THE
STUDENT NURSE HANDBOOK

A
SURVIVAL
GUIDE

Your textbook comes with a range of additional online resources

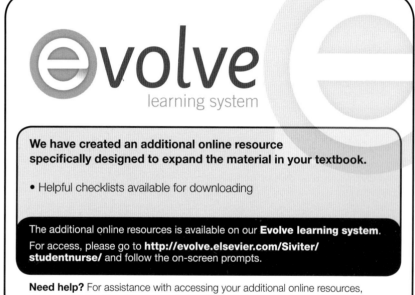

evolve
learning system

We have created an additional online resource specifically designed to expand the material in your textbook.

• Helpful checklists available for downloading

The additional online resources is available on our **Evolve learning system**.
For access, please go to **http://evolve.elsevier.com/Siviter/studentnurse/** and follow the on-screen prompts.

Need help? For assistance with accessing your additional online resources, please visit **http://evolvesupport.elsevier.com/**

Content Strategist: Mairi McCubbin
Content Development Specialist: Sheila Black
Project Manager: Lucía Pérez
Designer: Miles Hitchen

THE
STUDENT
NURSE
HANDBOOK

A SURVIVAL GUIDE

Third Edition

Bethann Siviter BSc(Hons) Dip(HE) RN SPDN

Consultant Nurse

Past Chair of the RCN Association of Nursing Students

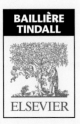

BAILLIÈRE
TINDALL

ELSEVIER

Edinburgh   London   New York   Oxford
Philadelphia   St Louis   Sydney   Toronto 2013

BAILLIÈRE
TINDALL
ELSEVIER

© 2013 Elsevier Ltd. All rights reserved.

First edition 2004
Second edition 2008
Third edition 2013

ISBN 978-0-7020-4579-0

British Library Cataloguing in Publication Data
A catalogue record for this book is available from the British Library

Library of Congress Cataloging in Publication Data
A catalog record for this book is available from the Library of Congress

 your source for books,
journals and multimedia
in the health sciences
www.elsevierhealth.com

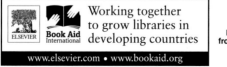

Working together
to grow libraries in
developing countries

www.elsevier.com • www.bookaid.org

The
Publisher's
policy is to use
**paper manufactured
from sustainable forests**

Printed in China

Contents

Preface   ix
Acknowledgements   xi

1 Becoming and Being a Nurse   1

What is nursing?   2
The NMC   5
What kinds of jobs and career paths can start
with nursing?   12
Who can become a nurse?   18
What are the paths to becoming a nurse?   20
Choosing your university   22
I have got on to a course – now what happens?   23
FAQ   25
References   26
Contacts   26

2 Nursing Models   29

Nursing   31
Nursing process   32
Holism   33
Philosophy   35
Transcultural care   36
Family-based care   36
Nursing theory   36
Framework   37
Models   37
Assessing yourself   50
References   52

3 Academic Work   54

Referencing   55
Plagiarism   56
Writing an assignment   58
Confidentiality and privacy   64
Basic IT skills   66
References   67
Assignment information worksheet   68

4 Clinical Placements 69

Nurse education changes in the late twentieth century 70
The Peach Report 70
Making a difference 71
The branches of nursing 72
Clinical placements 73
Supernumerary status 79
Becoming a nurse one placement at a time 81
Mentorship 81
Other people who help you learn 83
References 86
Clinical placement checklist 87

5 Basics of Nursing 89

Basic nursing qualities 89
Vignettes 90
Communication skills 93

6 Tools of the Trade 100

Assertiveness 100
Boundaries 104
Coping with stress 106
Delegation and organization 108
Ethics 112
Leadership 116
Norms 118
Governance 119
Standards: Essence of care and standards
for better health 121
References 122

7 Cracking the Code 123

Introduction to the language of nurses 123
Nursing/medical jargon 124
Medical terminology in general 126
Anatomical positions and descriptions 127
Word root basics 129
Common suffixes and prefixes 130

8 Safe and Accurate Administration of Medicines   131

Medication errors   *131*
Safe and responsible administration of medication   *132*
Nursing responsibilities   *136*
Numeracy   *138*
Dosage calculations   *141*
References   *152*

9 Reading and Understanding Research   153

Why is research important to evidence-based practice?   *154*
Research basics   *156*
Reading research critically   *157*
Applying research to practice   *163*
The power of research   *163*
Approaching research   *166*
Writing a research proposal   *166*

10 Reflective Practice and Portfolios   171

What is reflection?   *171*
Reflective models   *173*
Why reflection is important to practice   *174*
Portfolios   *175*
References   *179*

11 Legal Issues for Students   180

Records and record-keeping   *181*
Disability and the Disability Discrimination Act (NI)
    or Equality Act (GB)   *183*
The Data Protection Act   *186*
The Health and Safety at Work Act   *187*
Duty of care   *189*
Consent   *190*
Accountability   *192*
Fitness for practice   *192*
Negligence   *193*
Bullying   *194*
The Mental Capacity Act   *195*
References   *198*

Final Thoughts	199
Useful Books, Journals and Other Resources	201
Appendices:	
Appendix 1: The National Union of Students - NUS	207
Appendix 2: Nursing and Midwifery Council (NMC) Standards for Pre-Registration Nursing Education (2010)	210
Appendix 3: Tips for Mental Health Nursing	212
Appendix 4: Learning Disabilities Nursing	216
Appendix 5: Tips for Children's Nursing	224
Appendix 6: Nursing Older People	226
Appendix 7: Knowledge and Skills Framework	228
Appendix 8: Root Words, Prefixes and Suffixes	231
Appendix 9: Normal Values	240
Index	244

Preface

The first edition of the Student Nurse Handbook was written while I was still a student myself, in a District Nursing BSc(Hons) course I undertook on the heels of my Dip(HE). The second edition was written while I was recovering from the course of events that led to me becoming disabled. To be honest, it's nice to start this edition without any difficult event or overwhelming commitment looming!

As with the second edition, I had to make sure that a nurse many years on from qualification would be a suitable person to write this book for beginners: was it time for someone else to take this book forward? I had to admit that I could no more give up this book and its connection to students than give up nursing: being here for you is important to me.

I have become established in practice and in advocacy for disabled people and disability rights, but central to my heart remains the desire to help nurses and nursing students to become the kind of nurse patients need, as well as to enjoy the many personal rewards nursing can bring. I love that special fresh-faced enthusiasm, that desire to learn and patient-focused passion for caring and nursing itself that nursing students always seem to have. I find myself refreshed and rejuvenated after being with students, and so, again, I am here with this book, feeling both grateful for a chance to support you and energized by the exercise. As with the first two editions, I want this book to be a knowing friend, to encourage you, help you and get you through the course and into a nursing post.

The information in the Handbook has been refreshed and updated to bring it in line with the pre-registration nursing review held by the NMC and the changes nurse education is facing. I have been involved in that review; I stood for a place on the NMC's Professional Practice and Registration Committee, so I could support students as much as possible, and I know some of the things that students brought to me as concerns have been resolved through the review.

I hope this new edition gives you what you need. I am not perfect: if I have made mistakes, I am sorry – please tell us so we can fix them. Please also tell us what you liked. Know that on every page I am there with you, as a friend who has been there too, but who also knows what rewards and challenges await.

There is a saying on my office wall *'What you experience in life, no one can take away from you'* – this is critical for a nurse to remember. Nurse education converts you into a new person – you see the world differently and use a different framework for decisions; you are forever a 'nurse'. The kind of nurse you become depends not simply on your experiences, but also on how you process and learn from them. Continue to grow and learn, and you will always be fascinated and excited by nursing and its opportunities, always ready to rise to the challenge each patient presents, to deliver with kindness and compassion the nursing care they need. Be a role model for reflection and for patient-focused care; show others that you put patients first and are willing to evolve as a nurse.

The years of your course will pass whether you are in nursing education or not – take advantage of the time, no matter how challenging, and become the nurse you want and need to be.

Give your family and friends a break – they don't understand what is happening to you; they want to help you and don't know how. Don't lose track of people – relationships suffer when you are in Nurse Education, so make sure to give some time to family and friends, and don't spend it all talking about nursing . . . it will do you a world of good. Try to not kill yourself working too many hours: there will be plenty of time for hard work once you qualify. Get together with like-minded students, and don't be afraid to speak up if things are not as they should be. Welcome to the wonderful world of nursing!

Birmingham, 2013   *Bethann Siviter*

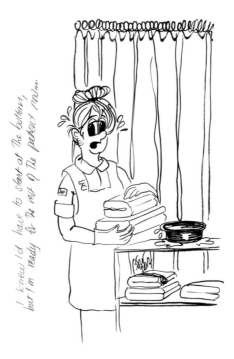

Acknowledgements

I have some very special people and one exceptionally special 'non-person' to thank. These people are my very special heroes and inspirations, who have all, in their own way, made my life so very special.

In addition to my husband Andrew, who is my best friend, carer, partner and everything else, my 'sister', Helen, and nephew, Oliver, for picking up the pieces so many times, and my friend Sue Evans for teaching me more about myself than I sometimes wished to know, I would like to thank:

- Canine Partners (www.caninepartners.org.uk), as an organization and group of fantastic people who provided me with my assistance dog and all the training I needed to make it work. So many of the staff have been so supportive I cannot name them all, but they know.

- Taska, my Black Labrador assistance dog and constant helpful companion, who has patiently given me silent encouragement and active help in every aspect of life . . . she is an amazing friend and companion, and I cannot imagine life without her.

- Jan and Richard Hirons, who raised Taska for Canine Partners, giving her 14 months of love and training only to give her up, knowing that someone disabled needed her but not knowing if they would ever see her again. I am so grateful for the dog you created.

- Leona McCarthy, for loving Taska as much as I do, and giving her the training she needed to prove what a worthy girl she is. Thank you for understanding me and Taz. Leona, you are a friend I shall never forget – and neither will Taska.

- Julia Hurley, for giving me all the help, advocacy and support I needed, which was far more than I deserved. Your patience and understanding give me so much confidence – and your tolerance got me through some of the most challenging moments of my time with Taz.

- To all the Canine Partners family who have given so much encouragement and help . . . what a loving bunch of people.

And finally, thanks to Stella Hewitt and her faithful Canine Partner, Jenson, without whose loving support there would have been no Taska. Without Stella, who is herself disabled, the money to pay for Taska and her training would have remained in the various pockets across the country from which Stella so gracefully coaxed it through her Colour Wheel Appeal. Stella, you may not be a nurse, but you are a healer, and I am forever grateful.

Becoming and Being a Nurse

> ❝Nursing is doing for others what they would do for themselves, if they had the knowledge and ability. It's also about thinking, not filling out forms, but about knowing the kinds of things most people need and anticipating their needs without being told. A nurse who can't think isn't a nurse. I hate it that our Model has become a paperwork exercise – nurses need brains to guide their practice, not paper. . .❞
>
> *Nancy Roper*

In this chapter

- What is nursing?
- The NMC
- What kinds of jobs and career paths can start with nursing?
- Who can become a nurse?
- What are the paths to becoming a nurse?
- Choosing your university
- I have got on to a course – now what happens?
- FAQs
- References

In Chapters 5 (Basics of Nursing) and 6 (Tools of the Trade) you will find concrete skills essential for nursing.

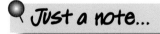

Just a note...

When I speak about nurses, I use female pronouns – this is not as a judgement about men as nurses (I feel gender is irrelevant as a basic nursing qualification) but to avoid confusion and the bulky he/she/his/hers syntax. Men are valued and play an important role in nursing.

WHAT IS NURSING?

Nursing defined

In 1966, Virginia Henderson, a nursing theorist, wrote:

> Nursing is primarily assisting the individual in their performance of those activities contributing to health, or its recovery that they would perform unaided if they had the necessary strength, will, or knowledge.

The Royal College of Nursing (2003) has defined nursing as:

> The use of clinical judgement in the provision of care to enable people to improve, maintain, or recover health, to cope with health problems, and to achieve the best possible quality of life, whatever their disease or disability, until death.

What these definitions have in common is that nurses:

- use clinical judgement, which requires education and experience
- help people who are well to stay well
- help people who are ill to get better
- help people who won't get better to have the best life possible
- do for people what they would do for themselves
- promote good health
- provide care and services
- help people to cope with problems and concerns
- help many different people of different ages with many different problems
- help and support the families and carers of people receiving nursing care.

Nancy's quote at the beginning of this chapter really sits at the heart of nursing practice: nurses need to know what their patients will need, anticipate what kinds of help they will require, and do what is needed without anyone telling them to. You may feel that even as a student your nursing life is filled with documents and paperwork, but a nurse should use the paperwork as a tool, not find that the paperwork uses *her*. In a minute, I will explain why the paperwork is so overwhelming.

Nursing heroes

To be inspired by some of the many nursing heroes who have preceded you, you might want to look up a few of the following famous names: Florence Nightingale, Mary Seacole, Elizabeth Nneka Anionwu, Ethel Gordon Fenwick, Edith Louisa Cavell, Rufaida Al Aslamiya and Nancy Roper (as in Roper Logan and Tierney).

There are countless nursing heroes – many without recognized names, people who work lousy hours in difficult jobs to make sure that those who need them have good care. Whether on the battlefield or in the inner city, working with children or older people, nurses have a special job – bringing health to those who need them. You are one of many, and in your profession you have the opportunity to be a real hero to those for whom you care. Look for inspiration in nursing history, but also in the nurses around you.

Vocation vs profession: the evolution of nursing

Nursing is a profession; when it started, it was considered a 'vocation'. A vocation implies a sense of 'calling', as for those in religious life. It implies that some people are 'born to be nurses' because of certain personal qualities fundamental to nursing. A profession implies that nursing can be learned, because learning theory and knowledge makes one a nurse. Personally, I think aspects of vocation are essential in nursing – it takes a lot to be patient, kind and compassionate all the time, even when your feet hurt, you missed lunch (again) and you (still) haven't got enough time to pee. They can't teach that kind of selflessness in university, and if the world was perfect we wouldn't have to work so hard – but it's not perfect, so we need to be something special or our patients will suffer. You can decide to develop the kinds of skills we once thought needed to be inborn, and you can keep them, but to do that your choice must always be forefront in your mind. Your patient has to come first, every minute of every day.

Nursing has changed a lot – but that will never change. If you want to be the kind of nurse patients need, your comfort must come second. That doesn't mean you should be abused; it just means that if it's lunchtime and one of you has to wait for lunch, it shouldn't be your patient.

New pre-registration standards

It was in response to the chaos of problematic nursing practice that the NMC developed new standards for pre-registration nursing. One of the absolute premises underpinning the new standards was that while developing as professionals, we as nurses would not leave nursing behind: nursing needed to be rooted in compassion, kindness, caring and other vocational-style values while also giving new nurses a solid theoretical, practical and professional nursing-skill base. You will study under this new curriculum . . . but your mentor, and the nurses you work with, may have trained under a very different system. You may need to be an ambassador for the 'new old nursing', and the return to the essential values that are fundamental to nursing practice. These fundamentals are evident in the kinds of comments the public made when feeding into the consultation about the new nursing course:

> 'I want a nurse who I feel safe with, who is kind, gentle and who knows what to do ... '
>
> 'Nurses need to smile, be patient, and not give us infections because they didn't wash their hands ... '
>
> 'We want our angels back ... the ones who made us comfortable, who put us first – where have they gone?'

These are examples of the kinds of comments the public made – loud and clear, they told the NMC they wanted both a vocational and a professional nurse.

Embedding these standards in the new course took a lot of groundwork. New expectations for nurses who would serve as mentors, increased accountability for mentors, and more information about standards in practice were planned to work together to give nursing a better footing. Something else happened in the new course, too – for the first time, reasonable adjustments for students with disabilities were written into the standards, both for academic and placement environments. Nursing was becoming more accessible to those who might previously have been shut out. Other changes were also made – multidisciplinary placements, increased community exposure, clear criteria for progression throughout the course, involvement of service users and carers, an improved common foundation that allowed every nurse to provide a basic level of care no matter which field of nursing they come from, and a better foundation for specialist practice. There are clear, universal outcomes where every student across the UK will have to achieve at the same minimum level in order to qualify.

The course will give you information about the standards and what you are expected to achieve; not only will you need to show that you understand and can apply theory and achieve essential skills, you will also need to prove that you can provide compassionate, kind and patient-centred care. Isn't that why you came into nursing in the first place? Look on the NMC website for information and an outline of the NMC pre-registration standards.

Included in the standards are essential skills clusters – groups of skills the student will need to develop to qualify. These are offered at increasing levels of complexity and responsbility, so students can demonstrate their increasing proficiency. Whereas in previous programmes each placement had its own assessment, the new course uses one connected assessment process – instead of placements being islands, they are now pulled together so that not only is the student journey better supported, but students' achievement (or failure to achieve) over the entire course is also more obvious.

I was honoured to serve on the NMC committee (Professional Practice and Registration) that developed the pre-registration standards, and believe they are the best thing to happen to nurse education. I sincerely hope they will give you what you need to be the nurse you came into nursing to be.

Nursing as a career

As you develop as a nurse, nursing will become part of you and will guide the way you think and act in every situation, not just at work. Some people jokingly say that becoming a nurse is a terminal disease – the way you see the world, and people in it, will be coloured by your nursing knowledge and judgement for the rest of your life. You will never again be able to see the world uncoloured by your knowledge about people, health, social issues, psychology and the way healthcare is delivered. You will hear someone cough, and think 'Do they have a cold or an obstructed airway?'; you will criticize *Holby City*, *Casualty* and similar shows, and suddenly no one except other nursing students will share a meal with you because you will talk about body fluids and function over food. So stepping into nursing is not just entering a profession – it's allowing the profession to enter you. You might leave nursing and have other careers, but what you learn as a nurse will always be a part of you. Nursing has evolved and must continue to do so – and you, as a nurse, must be prepared to evolve and grow too.

THE NMC

What is the NMC?

The NMC is here to protect the public . . .

NMC website

> The NMC guides nurses to improve their practice, not only by telling them that they will get into trouble if they practise badly, but by explaining what patients need. The NMC really is one of nursing's greatest protectors, by setting limits and saying "to be a nurse, you must uphold certain standards . . ." they protect the public, but they also protect nursing.
>
> *New nurse*

> The NMC are there to keep nursing focused. They aren't looking for bad nurses so they can stomp on them – they are looking to make sure they help nurses be the right kind of nurses.
>
> *Student nurse, Year 3*

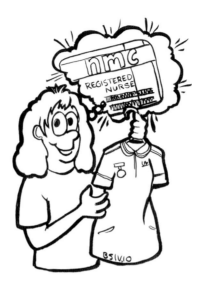

The Nursing and Midwifery Council (NMC) is an organization that ensures nurses, midwives and health visitors provide high standards of care to their patients and clients. At some point, it may even regulate healthcare support workers. It is governed by a combination of lay (non-nursing) members and nursing practitioners, working together to make decisions, set out policy and determine the direction the NMC should take. Every nurse can apply to work with the NMC on committees and working groups, working in partnership with the regulator and the public to shape nursing.

Qualified nurses, midwives and health visitors are registered through the NMC, and the NMC has the right to suspend or remove practitioners from the register if it is proven that the practitioner is not safe, or does not behave in a professional manner. But the NMC doesn't see its role as 'Profession Police'– the NMC sees itself as a partner in practice, helping the nurse to live up to the demands of nursing without letting the patient down.

The NMC also sets out criteria for education and practice, gives advice to nurses, midwives and health visitors, and publishes numerous publications to support good practice. You know how much impact the new Pre-registration Standards for Nursing Students has had. Among the NMC publications you will find most useful are the *Code of Professional Conduct* and the *Guide for Students of Nursing and Midwifery*. Please read them and refer back to them during your course. You can search the NMC website (www.nmc-uk.org) for information on many different subjects. Most of the NMC or UKCC publications are available on this website as a document file, or can be posted to you on request.

Before the NMC, the United Kingdom Central Council (UKCC) had these responsibilities. There was a national board in each of the four UK countries, which worked with the UKCC; these national boards have now been disbanded and, together with the UKCC, have become the NMC. There may come a time when the NMC evolves into another organization; there is currently a suggestion that nurses should perhaps not regulate themselves – that instead of being governed by a body including nurses they should be governed by central government. However, nurses, and their professional organizations and trade unions, feel strongly that it is essential for nurses to govern nursing.

The one document with which most nurses are familiar is the NMC *Code of Professional Conduct*. This a 'rulebook' for nursing, midwifery and health visiting – it tells you what is expected of you and what you should expect of others, and it highlights the criteria against which you will be measured should there ever be a complaint about your practice.

When writing an assignment or a reflection, always try to find where the NMC Code fits in and cite it. It proves that you are aware of, and paying attention to, the guidelines set out for safe and competent practice. It will help you to get good marks and become a responsible nurse. Also, use the NMC Code when you are making decisions in your clinical area. The entire Code is very long, but don't be intimidated. The basic points are that, as a registered nurse, midwife or health visitor, you must:

- respect the patient or client as an individual
- obtain consent before you give any treatment or care
- cooperate with others in the team
- protect confidential information
- maintain your professional knowledge and competence
- be trustworthy
- act to identify and minimize the risk to patients and clients.

The NMC *Guide for Students of Nursing and Midwifery* is very easy to read, and really gives you important information and support. It explains how the Code of Conduct applies to you, and how you are expected to act as a student nurse. These two documents are included in this chapter to highlight how important they are if you are to become a safe and competent practitioner. I cannot over-emphasize how much these documents can help you in your course. The main points of the NMC *Guide for Students of Nursing and Midwifery* are that:

- you must always work under the supervision of a qualified nurse or midwife, as you are not accountable under the NMC *Code of Professional Conduct*. You are, however, responsible for working within the limitations of your role as a student.
- you must always identify yourself as a student nurse. You must always let patients and their families know that you are a student, and you must

identify yourself as a student on the telephone. Patients have a right to say 'No' to a student caring for them.

- you have an obligation to maintain patient confidentiality.
- you must never do *anything* that is outside your role as a student.

When you finish your course (and, yes – there is light at the end of the nursing education tunnel!) you will register with the NMC. The way it currently works is:

1.   You successfully finish your course (thinking ' . . . and am I glad I had the *Student Nurse Handbook* . . . ').
2.   Your uni sends the NMC a list of graduates and affirms that you, as individuals, are of 'good character'. This declaration is an essential part of your process to join the register (don't worry: if there are any concerns, you will know about them before it gets to this point). Make absolutely certain that your uni spells your name properly and sends the NMC your current address.
3.   The NMC sends your registering information, asks you to confirm your name and address, and tells you where to send the registration fee. Remember: if someone else is paying your fees for you, make sure your name, address and NMC personal identification number (PIN) are on the cheque.
4.   You wait. Registration doesn't take as long as it used to, but the wait is still nerve-wracking. You have waited all this time to be a real nurse, and you ache to wear the blue uniform . . . and get the nurse's pay! Although you will probably be paid as an HCA while you are waiting for your PIN to be added to the register, most employers pay you the higher rate retrospectively once it comes through. Remember: you cannot call yourself a nurse until your PIN is registered.
5.   When your PIN comes through, call your employers and let them know. They have a special contact at the NMC to confirm your registration.

Something to think about: now you are earning, clothes, a car – all those things that have been waiting while you were a student – are suddenly within your reach. It will also be very easy to get credit. The joy of finishing your course, getting a real job and finally being a nurse can mute your common sense a bit, so don't get ahead of yourself and spend all your money!

When your PIN comes through, you are a card-carrying nurse. You are now accountable under the *Code of Professional Conduct* and, in the not-too-distant future, a student nurse will be working with you, looking up to you and wondering, 'Will I ever be able to do what she does?', just like you did with your mentor. Please don't get qualified-nurse amnesia: never forget what it was like to be a student. You know how frustrating and stressful it is; you know what a difference a good and interested mentor can make. If you had bad mentors, the best way to make up for it is always to be a good one.

Once you become a nurse, the NMC is there for you – for advice, for information, for guidance, and for documents and publications to guide your practice. It is also the body that will make a decision about your fitness to practise should a question ever arise. If you are convicted of a crime or if there is an allegation that your practice does not meet the required standard – for any reason – it can go to the NMC for consideration.

If you want to know what happens when the NMC looks at your practice, you can look at what has happened to others. You can go and attend a disciplinary hearing, but this might be too intense. You can also go to the NMC website (www.nmc-uk.org) and look at 'fitness to practise', where you can see the outcomes of hearings. You will see that you *can* be struck off – lose your right to practise as a nurse – for such things as poor documentation, poor care, even impatience. Your status as a nurse relies on you maintaining standards – so when you are trying to follow the Code and a nurse says to you 'yes, but in the real world . . . ', remember that in the real world there are fitness-to-practise hearings, where the NMC is looking at what you did . . . and if you fail to meet your obligations under the Code, you will no longer be a nurse.

If you are willing to work hard for 3 years or more to become a nurse, don't let a slip take it all away. Make a commitment to be the kind of nurse patients need; the NMC will help you if you ask. Don't let yourself become one of those many nurses who let things slide. In the 'real world', you are expected to maintain high standards. If any nurse expects you to cut corners, ask her what she knows about fitness-to-practise hearings at the NMC. Nothing terrifies a nurse more than being found guilty of misconduct and being struck off: why chance it when there are ways to avoid it completely? All you have to do is follow the Code of Conduct: simple.

The Code of Practice: May 2008

The code is the foundation of your practice, and essential for public wellbeing. It gives you guidance, but also sets out the boundaries for your practice and your behaviour as a person and professional.

In the most basic terms, the code says that 'the people in your care must be able to trust you with their health and wellbeing.' It then goes on to explain what you must do to be worthy of that trust. You must:

- put your patients first, treating them with respect and dignity as unique people who have a right to live as they choose, but also to get the help they need.
- work with others, in healthcare and social care, to make sure that everyone has better health and wellbeing – be vigilant regarding public health issues and be an advocate for health

- be aware of your responsibilities, and the evidence behind practice so you can show that what you do is the right thing . . . your standards must be high, because your patients deserve the best.
- be a person who acts ethically and lawfully, with personal and professional integrity, and who is seen as the kind of nurse that a nurse should be.
- be accountable for what you do and what you fail to do, and be able to explain the rationale behind your actions. You must learn to make good decisions, based on both objective and subjective assessments, but you must also avoid being biased or judging people. You must continue to work and develop, and never take for granted that you can do the right thing – you must stop and think, being certain that you are skilled and knowledgeable.
- act with knowledge and skill, but also with kindness and compassion. You must never say or do anything that causes your patient unnecessary stress or pain. You must put your patient, their needs and preferences, and the input of their family and carers, first.

The register

When you qualify as a nurse, you are placed on the register – a list of all those who are qualified to work as nurses throughout the UK. In addition to your basic nursing qualification in the branch in which you studied, there are additional registerable qualifications: specialist practice, teaching, and nurse prescribing. The list of recordable qualifications may change, but for now, those qualifications listed here are the only ones.

There are different categories of the register. Level 1 nurses are Registered Nurses trained in one of the Fields of Practice (branches). Level 2 nurses are Enrolled Nurses, and nurses can no longer 'enroll' as nurses. Although Level 2 nurses are registered nurses, too, they need to upgrade to Level 1 to develop specialist practice or usually to go beyond Band 5. Don't confuse second level with second class – many Level 2 nurses are top-notch, and all had a gruelling, demanding training preparing them to deliver practical nursing care. These nurses are skilled and knowledgeable practitioners and are experts in the delivery of hands-on care. Don't underestimate their knowledge and experience. In the USA, these nurses are called LPN or LVN (Licensed Practice or License Vocational Nurses).

The terms and abbreviations used on the register have changed, because the register changed in 2007. The following table shows the evolution of nursing qualifications, along with the letters which these qualifications entitle you to use after your name. For example, I am Bethann Siviter, BSc(Hons), RNA, SPDN, V100, DipHE. I use 'RNA' because even though I qualified before 2007, my qualification was converted to the new register. It might be helpful for you to see the different qualifications and names we nurses have used . . .

Nursing Qualifications pre-2007
These are only used by those who qualified before the new Register in 2007.

State Registered Nurse (before 1984)	SRN
Registered General Nurse (after 1984)	RGN
Registered Mental Health Nurse	RMN
Registered Sick Children's Nurse	RSCN
State Enrolled Nurse (before 1984)	SEN
State Enrolled Nurse (Mental Illness) (before 1984)	SEN(M)
Enrolled Nurse (after 1984)	EN
Enrolled Nurse (Mental Illness) (after 1984)	EN(M)
Registered Nurse Mental Handicapped	RNMH
Registered Nurse (qualified nurse)	RN

Nursing and Midwifery Qualifications on the New Register

Registered Midwife	RM
1st Level Registered Nurse (Adult)	RN1 / RNA
2nd Level Registered Nurse (Adult) (previously Enrolled Nurse)	RN2
1st Level Registered Nurse (Mental Health)	RN3 / RNMH
2nd Level Registered Nurse (Mental Health) (previously Enrolled Nurse, Mental Illness)	RN4
1st Level Registered Nurse (Learning Disabilities)	RN5 / RNLD
2nd Level Registered Nurse (Learning Disabilities)	RN6
1st Level Registered Nurse (Children)	RN8 / RNC
2nd Level Registered Nurse (General)	RN7
2nd Level Registered Nurse (Fever)	RN9
Specialist Community Public Health Nurse (Health Visiting)	RHV
Specialist Community Public Health Nurse (School Nursing)	RSN
Specialist Community Public Health Nurse (Occupational Health)	ROH
Specialist Community Public Health Nurse (Family Health Nursing) (Scotland Only)	RFHN

Recorded Qualifications
These are additional qualifications that are added once you are already on the register as a Level 1 nurse. The NMC guidance for achievement underpins the courses, so that nurses can register their recorded qualifications.

Specialist Practitioner – Adult Nursing	SPAN
Specialist Practitioner – Mental Health Nursing	SPMH
Specialist Practitioner – Children's Nursing	SPCN
Specialist Practitioner – Learning Disability Nursing	SPLD
Specialist Practitioner – General Practice Nursing	SPGP
Specialist Practitioner – Community Mental Health Nursing	SCHM
Specialist Practitioner – Community Learning Disabilities Nursing	SCLD
Specialist Practitioner – Community Children's Nursing	SPCC
Specialist Practitioner – District Nursing	SPDN
Mode 1 Prescribing	V100
Extended Nurse Prescribing	V200
Extended/Supplementary Nurse Prescribing	V300
Lecturer/Practice Educator	LPE

Public Health Practitioners – nurses who have specialist education and qualification in one of the following areas – are registered in the Specialist Community Public Health (SCPH) part of the register:

- Health Visitor
- School Nurse

- Occupational Health Nurse
- Family Health (Scotland).

Every year, you pay to stay on the register; every 3 years, you need to prove that you have remained up to date in your practice. There will be increasingly formal processes for nurses to prove that they continue to be fit to practise.

WHAT KINDS OF JOBS AND CAREER PATHS CAN START WITH NURSING?

As a nurse, you can work in many different areas and with many different people. There are now four different basic branches in nursing. During your pre-registration course you can become:

- a children's nurse
- an adult nurse
- a learning disability nurse
- a mental health nurse.

You will need to choose, usually when you apply, which branch of nursing you want to enter. If you are really unhappy, or find yourself very interested in another branch, you may be able to change – but the sooner you do this, the easier it will be.

Becoming an advanced nurse starts with basic nursing – for example, to be become a school nurse you need a background in children's nursing. It is important that you identify the path to where you want to be: it is not always possible to get to a certain career if you haven't taken the correct branch. In the following list, if it is more helpful to follow one branch over another I will try to let you know.

Nursing is the foundation for a number of careers and pathways – some are direct advancements of your nursing career, like being a nurse manager, but, some, like midwifery, are new careers requiring additional education and preparation; although these careers might be related to nursing they are *not* nursing in and of themselves. This list includes some ideas for those who want to enter nursing but who also want to know what the future might hold for them, and also jobs that people may have while working to become a nurse.

- **Midwife**: midwives care for pregnant women, and deliver and care for babies. You can become a midwife without being a nurse, or you can take a midwifery course after becoming a nurse. It's a complex and demanding profession that is independent from nursing. If it's really your life's desire to become a midwife, apply first to a midwifery course. The transition from nurse to midwife can be difficult for some, as permission to enter the course can be affected by workforce needs, such as a shortage of nurses needed in other areas. Although a nurse can enter midwifery studies, this is a different qualification; having a background in women's health or children's nursing is helpful, but not required. British midwives have a worldwide reputation for excellence. Check out the Royal College of Midwives for more information (www.rcm.org.uk).

- **Health visitor**: health visitors (HVs) help new mothers and teach them how to care for their children, help those children to be healthy, and/or promote good health for families. They have an essential role in child protection and work closely with social workers, midwives, learning disability and children's nurses, as well as with other nurses and professionals to maintain good public health and safety. Becoming a health visitor requires an additional post-basic qualification at degree or postgraduate diploma level. A health visitor currently trains as a nurse first, and joins the Specialist Public Health part of the register when she becomes a health visitor (as a result of specialist degree-level education); at some point in the future, a person may train specifically to be a health visitor and not train as a nurse at all. Health visitors have a special place and a special category in the nursing register; their specialty in health promotion, health education and health improvement is reflected in their title – Specialist Public Health nurses.

- **Children's nurse**: children's nurses are specialists in the health and care of children, and can work in any area of care where there are children. Children's nursing is one of the basic pre-registration nursing branches. A nurse registered as a children's nurse can use the letters RNC after her name.

- **Adult nurse**: adult nurses work in the community, in hospitals, in care homes, clinics, etc., and are specially prepared for the care and support of people from early adulthood to old age in a variety of settings. Adult nursing is one of the basic pre-registration branches. (Although it's not really the same as Adult branch nursing, someone who specifies a 'registered general nurse' (RGN) usually means an Adult-branch registered nurse – historically the generically trained nurse was called an RGN, and the others were specialists, so the name has stuck to the Adult branch nurse). A nurse registered as an adult nurse can use the letters RNA after her name.

- **Learning disability nurse**: learning disability nurses are specialists in caring for and meeting the needs of people with learning disabilities, and can work in a hospital, care home or school, or in a patient's home – wherever there is a client with special needs. Learning disability nursing is one of the basic pre-registration branches. A nurse registered as a learning disability nurse can use the letters RNLD after her name.

- **Mental health nurse**: mental health nurses specialize in the care and support of people with mental illness, and can work in any setting where there are clients. Mental health nursing is one of the basic pre-registration branches. One mistake that people make is calling one of these nurses a 'mental' nurse; this sounds disparaging and judgemental, so stick to 'mental health nurse'. A nurse registered as a mental health nurse can use the letters RNMH after her name.

- **School nurse**: school nurses promote health and support children in school. They often work very closely with health visitors, and undertake a substantial health promotion and health education role. Registration as a school nurse is a specialist practice area requiring degree-level or postgraduate education. A background in children's nursing is common for nurses who become school nurses.

- **Occupational health nurse**: occupational health nurses protect and care for people at work. They do first aid, offer counselling on stress, promote healthy practices at home and at work, and help employers keep their employees healthy. Being an occupational health nurse requires a post-basic qualification at postgraduate diploma or degree level, and registration on a Specialist Practice part of the register. Usually, nurses who have qualified as an RNA enter occupational health nursing.

- **District nurse**: district nurses care for people in their homes. They have a very broad specialty, including wound care, continence and care of chronically ill patients. They work closely with other nurses and other professionals to deliver care and provide support for people who are either too ill to leave their homes, or have such significant mobility problems that they are unable to do so easily. Being a district nurse requires a post-basic qualification at postgraduate diploma or degree level, and the qualification is considered a specialist practice part of the register. Usually, nurses who have qualified as an RNA enter district nursing.

- **Practice nurse**: practice nurses (PNs) work in a GP surgery, seeing patients with ongoing problems like asthma or diabetes, doing dressing changes and wound care, giving immunizations and health advice. Practice nurses, like district nurses, work closely with many other nurses and professionals. Being a practice nurse requires a post-basic qualification at postgraduate diploma or degree level, and usually it is nurses who have qualified as an RNA who enter this career path.

- **Research nurse**: research nurses carry out the research to provide evidence for nursing care. Most research nurses will have specialist education and/or a degree. Depending on the area of research, a nurse from any branch can become a research nurse.

- **Nurse educator**: nurse educators teach both new nurses and nurses learning more advanced practice. They come at all different levels, and some also continue to work as specialists in their own areas of nursing. Educators develop from all the branches in nursing (a good thing – without educators, there wouldn't be nurses!)

- **Specialist nurse**: specialist nurses work with specific groups of clients, like people with diabetes, cancer, or special problems like incontinence or chronic wounds. These specially trained nurses provide support and care for patients and their families while teaching and supporting other nurses. Some nurses, like Marie Curie or MacMillan nurses, are employed by charities to deliver specialist care. The branch (or field of practice) in which a person is trained and practises tends to influence the kind of specialist she becomes; nurses develop as a specialist as they work – for example, a children's nurse working with cancer sufferers might advance to become a specialist cancer nurse for children.

- **Nurse consultant**: nurse consultants are experts who provide care, advice and support, and also work to develop policy and working practices. These nurses usually have a Master's degree or higher, or have evidence of Master's degree-level thinking – meaning that they can come up with new ideas, think critically, show a high level of understanding and theoretical knowledge, and are able to understand the importance of and apply research to their pratice. These nurses will have proven expertise in a specific area of nursing, much as the spcialist nurse does. A nurse who qualified as an RNA might be a consultant for older people, where a RNC might work as a consultant for children with cancer.

- **Nurse practitioner**: nurse practitioners are highly skilled nurses who deliver an advanced level of care in a certain specialty, such as accident and emergency. These nurses are usually trained at Master's degree level, with specific skills in assessment and treatment as well as (usually) in prescribing. A nurse can come from any branch and develop into a nurse practitioner.

- **Prison nurse and forensic nurse**: nurses who work in a prison have a very demanding role – first aid, counselling and health promotion in a strict and sometimes dangerous environment. They need both mental health and general nursing skills. Forensic nurses usually have a mental health background. They provide care and ongoing assessment in hospitals and supervised environments, and sometimes even in the community, in situations where the patient has become involved with the court/legal system but needs care for a significant mental illness or learning disability. (Note that this is not to say that people with mental health issues or who are learning disabled are guilty of crime or should be seen as criminals; however, it is true that sometimes aspects of a mental illness or learning disability can contribute to a person becoming involved in the legal system – and if so, it is often a forensic nurse who can help them. Nurses don't judge people, they take care of them.) Some forensic nurses have an even wider scope, and offer support to victims of crime and criminal trauma as well. Prison and forensic nursing are different but have some similarities – usually the places in which they are found – which is why they are listed together. Although these are very demanding and sometimes dangerous areas of nursing, the clients often are very needy and good nursing skills can make a huge difference.

- **Manager**: nurses can also work in management, at any one of a number of levels – managing a ward, a specialty area, a clinic, or even a Trust. Nurses from any branch go into management. A nurse may be a clinical manager, meaning that she is involved in clinical processes, or work at a level of management that is not connected to clinical practice.

- **Matron**: a matron is a nurse with extensive experience and skill who acts as a supervisor and manager, promoting good practice and supporting the work of other nurses. Matrons can come from any branch. A matron's job is ensuring that standards are met and maintained.

- **Community psychiatric nurse**: community psychiatric nurses (CPNs) are mental health nurses who specialize in the care of people in the community. CPNs might visit patients in hospital, talk to people who are recently bereaved or who have recently suffered an emotional trauma, or follow clients with mental health needs. They usually are RNMH nurses.

- **Health care assistant/nurse auxiliary**: these caregivers help deliver patient care in nearly every environment in the NHS and healthcare system. Different meanings are sometimes given to the two terms (a nurse auxiliary (NA) might be considered to be a higher level than a health care assistant (HCA), or vice versa), and in some places HCAs do more than help with nursing tasks (e.g., an HCA in a GP's surgery may also do some clerical work). Many HCAs and NAs are very experienced and have a wide range of valuable skills. Just because they aren't nurses *per se* doesn't mean that they are not valuable and important members of the healthcare team. In this book, when I refer to HCAs I mean those in the HCA or NA role.

Clearly, there are as many different kinds of nurses as there are people who need nurses! There is no way I could list every type of nursing – there are countless opportunities for nurses to do work that they enjoy and that interests them. Some nurses work in the community, in or around doctors' surgeries. Some work in acute care, community or rehab hospitals, some work in old peoples' homes, some work in residential or nursing home care – wherever there are people who need help, there will be nurses.

Agenda for change

Banding

Each band has a body of pay increments, plus at least one gateway – a key achievement that must be reached to progress. If your pay reaches a point where a degree is required but you do not have one, you will not advance in pay until you have a degree or a new job. Band 5 has two gateways: the first comes during your first year, where you should be assessed at 6 months and 1 year into the post. This is called 'preceptorship', and is only there for newly qualified professionals starting in Band 5.

HCAs could be in Bands 1 through 3, with occasional highly trained HCAs or specialist support workers on Band 4.

Band 5 is the lowest band a qualified nurse will usually work on. In this band, someone is expected to have a degree or professional qualification. Newly qualified nurses will go on to Band 5 at the bottom step, and reach the first gateway after 6 months of practice ('The Preceptorship Period'). This period of 6 months is considered an integration period when you require more support. After the sixth month, you should go up to the real starting point of the band. You could stay in Band 5 for a number of years as a junior staff nurse or staff nurse. You can look online for the most up-to-date pay bands (search for 'Nurse Pay' and the year).

Band 6 is the band for more experienced nurses – usually the level sisters/charge nurses once were. A Band 6 nurse will do everything a Band 5 does, but can take more responsibility for the work of others, to help, assess, train and manage them.

Band 7 is a senior post, usually someone with a specialty or senior level role. This nurse would perhaps be a nurse specialist, ward manager, matron, etc.

Band 8 is broken into four categories: a, b, c and d. Band 8 is for nurses who are in specialist senior roles – perhaps consultant nurse, assistant directors, matrons of a large service, etc. It is not usual for a nurse to go above these bands.

KSF: Knowledge and Skills Framework

The KSF is a document that shows, based on your job description and AFC band, what you should know and what skills you need to do your job. It has some expectations you will need to meet at the beginning – some will come as you approach the gateway in your pay band. There are different dimensions: some, like safety, are core dimensions that belong to everyone in the NHS; others are present in some jobs and not others. Common dimensions for nurses are HWB6 and HWB7 – both of these raise expectations that the person in that job will be able to assess patients, plan their care and carry out appropriate treatments. There are different levels in each dimension; the most basic level requires you to have awareness, while the highest level expects you not only to do this yourself, but also to consider others and what they should be doing.

Although a Band 5 nurse and a Band 6 nurse may have the same dimensions at the same level, the dimensions will be interpreted differently – the expectations for a Band 6 nurse will always be higher than for a Band 5 nurse, those for a Band 7 higher than for a Band 6, etc.

The KSF works in two ways: first, to tell you what you should be doing, and second, to tell your employer what it should be training you to do. It is not about judging a person or limiting their income; it's about making sure they have the skills and knowledge to do their job, and that they are getting the training and support they need.

WHO CAN BECOME A NURSE?

- **Can you listen as well as talk, or are you at least willing to learn?** Much of nursing is less about physical skill and more about communicating and working with people. Your course will help you learn to be a good communicator, so even if you are really shy or quiet you can still learn to become a good nurse.

- **Can you take care of people without being prejudiced or biased?** As a nurse, you will care for criminals, people who abuse drugs or alcohol, people who don't speak English, people who have a different skin colour to yours, elderly and very young people, people with learning disabilities and mental illness, rich people, poor people, likeable people, people who aren't very likeable, clean people, smelly people . . . and you have to treat them all fairly and with respect.

- **Can you commit to a lifetime of keeping up to date?** Nursing isn't something you learn once and never go back to. Nurses have a commitment to keep their knowledge and skills current, and need to be willing to constantly be thinking about what to learn next.

- **Have you done GCSEs or A levels (or equivalent)?** On the application form, it will explain the minimums. Basically, you need five GCSEs or a certain level of national vocational qualification (NVQ). You can find out about the minimum requirements from the Nursing and Midwifery Council (NMC) and from NHS Careers (see Contacts section at the end of this chapter). Some universities want more than the minimum, so if you have your heart set on a particular place, speak to them. Even if you don't have the minimum, you can take the Access course (more on this below).

- **Do you enjoy being with people?** As a nurse, you will always be with people. You could be with them in person, over the phone, or in any one of a number of different environments. You could even become a research nurse! No matter how you like to work, there is a place in nursing for you!

- **Are you healthy?** OK, before you read this, can I say that 'health' means the optimal level of function a person can have, given any limitations, problems, or underlying disease? (If you use that, cite me!) For example, if you are in perfect health except that you have diabetes, as long as the diabetes is controlled, you are healthy. This is something to think about when you are considering nursing, as being healthy is important; you will need to complete a health clearance form when you apply. If you have a disability, don't worry that you can't become a nurse; that's not true. The DDA (Disability Discrimination Act in Northern Ireland) and Equality Act (in the rest of the UK) both make it clear that people should not be limited by their disabilities without good reason. You may be able, with the right support, to become a nurse. (I am working as a nurse and I am disabled, so I'm proof!) Ask to speak with the occupational health team when the time comes – don't give up, or let someone dissuade you, without talking to occupational health! People with dyslexia, depression and even missing an arm have successfully become nurses. It was once unthought of that a disabled person might be a nurse, but now anything is possible. Disabled people are only really *disabled* by the misperceptions of and limits and obstructions put on them by the world, in my opinion.

Dyslexia. The text to the right shows what text might look like to a person with dyslexia.

| The word sare n otsp aced cor rect ly |
| We spell wrds xaktle az tha snd to us |
| Sometimesallthelettersarepushedtogether |

Dyslexia isn't a mental illness; neither is it something that should prevent someone from becoming a nurse. There is more to people than how well they read . . . don't let dyslexia stop a good nurse. The biggest obstacle people with dyslexia face is ignorance. There is help; there are strategies to make things easier, and there is no evidence that says people with dyslexia are dim or intellectually challenged – in fact, often they are people of above average intellect! If you or someone you know is dyslexic, the university is obliged to help you because, under the Disability Discrimination Act, you are disabled and you have a right to achieve. No one can say you are not good enough simply based on your dyslexia.

- **Do you have any criminal convictions?** If you have been convicted of anything, you need to say so on your application form. Most universities ask everyone for a criminal records check anyway, and may ask for further information if you do have a problem in your past. They will take the circumstances into consideration, so it's best to be prepared for this and be totally honest – it's better to show that you learned from your mistakes than have the university think you are dishonest. Some types of conviction will make it very difficult to get into nurse education; if you are worried, talk to someone at the university before you apply.

As you can see, almost anyone can become a nurse if they really want to. You don't have to be a self-sacrificing angel of mercy to become a good nurse! Even if you don't have a strong academic background, or have had run-ins with the law, or have a disability, you might be able to become a nurse. Contact the groups at the end of this chapter for more information.

WHAT ARE THE PATHS TO BECOMING A NURSE?

If you are aged 14–19 (or maybe even a little older), you can go to www.stepintothenhs.nhs.uk to learn more about the NHS and the careers it can offer.

- **Degree.** Nursing is an all degree profession across the UK. It takes 3–4 years to become a nurse.

- **Access course.** You can also take the Access to Higher Education course (the 'Access course'), which equips adults who don't have formal qualifications like GCSEs or A levels, or who have been out of education for a while, with the skills and knowledge needed to enter higher education. The course for nursing is usually 1 year full time or 2 years part time, and involves useful courses like psychology, as well as learning how to study and take good notes.

- **Past experience.** Sometimes, past experience can count for you. You can contact any local university and ask about accrediting prior and experiential learning (APEL). APEL may only count once you have been accepted onto the course.

- **Basic minimum.** If you already have the basic minimum (five GCSEs, or equivalent, at C or above, including English and a science), you can apply. You will also need to have good basic IT skills (or be willing to work to develop them), good basic numeracy skills (or be willing to develop them), and the ability to study, write a paper, and present your ideas to other people (or be willing . . . you get the idea).

Funding

Following a recent review of NHS student support by the Department of Health in England, from September 2012 the funding arrangements will change. In addition to not having to pay tuition for the course, all new nursing students will be eligible for a £1000 grant, a means tested bursary and a reduced rate non-means tested maintenance loan, which will vary according to where students live (in/out of London, with/without parents) and the number of weeks yearly that they attend university. Further information is available from the Department of Health website.

Students on old funding schemes will remain on those schemes until they leave the course.

As well as the basics, students can apply for additional allowances if they meet the criteria (for disabled students and those with dependants), and can claim travel costs to placements if going to a placement is more costly than going to the university.

The NHS Business Services Authority can give you important information and support your applications for tuition, funding and grants. Find them on

Facebook or online (www.nhsbsa.nhs.uk). Other useful sites include NHS Careers (www.nhscareers.nhs.uk), and Cavell Nurses' Trust (www.cavellnursestrust.org) – a charity that can provide emergency support to nurses and students.

Students in England, Scotland, Wales and Northern Ireland have different funding. You need to ask your university about the specifics.

Usually, to be eligible for any support or funding, applicants must:

- have been ordinarily resident in the United Kingdom and Islands throughout the 3 years preceding the start of the academic year, *and*
- be ordinarily resident in any UK country on the start of the academic year, *and*
- be settled in the United Kingdom under the terms of the Immigration Act 1971 (in other words, you must be ordinarily resident here without being subject to any restriction on the period for which you may stay).

No matter what you receive, you will need to buy your own books and pay for accommodation. Your uniforms (if you need them) should be provided through the university. Some travel costs may be reimbursed; you will need to find the current guidelines by speaking to your university.

If you are an international student, you will need further information about fees and bursaries as well as student visas. Contact the University and Colleges Admissions Service (UCAS) for up-to-date information (see Contacts section).

I can't afford to live on the bursary . . .

Working as a health care assistant (HCA) in a hospital, or as a carer in a specialist area such as a learning disability or mental health setting, can be an avenue into nursing. Employers can 'second' (pronounced SEE-conned) employees into educational programmes that meet their workforce planning needs. This means that your employer pays for your education and pays you a salary while you are in university. You might or might not have to go back and work for that employer after you qualify. Some employers offer scholarships instead of secondments; this means that instead of remaining an employee (and being the responsibility of the employer), you will have your tuition paid and get a stipend and perhaps even a bursary. This approach to sending employees into education is still evolving – if you are employed in a healthcare setting, and you are preparing to enter nurse education, ask your Human Resources (Personnel) department what might be available.

Another option is to undertake your nurse education in the military. Contact a recruiter for further information. Military nursing students have more demands placed on them, but they also get a much higher level of financial support while they are students.

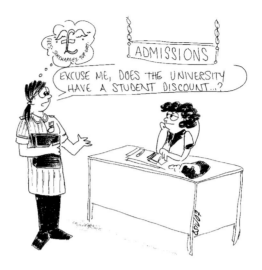

It is important that the economic disparity faced by nursing students is being addressed and hopefully soon those days will be gone where student nurses have to kill themselves working a full-time job on top of full-time education on top of the responsibilities of family life in order to survive economically until the end of the course. Contact the university in which you are most interested and ask them to explain student finance – they all have the information you will need. Please don't let worries about money prevent you from being a nurse – look forward to the financial rewards available once you qualify to help get you through.

OK, so you meet the entry requirements, have stocked up on baked beans and pot noodles, are ready to be skint for the next 3 or 4 years – now what?

CHOOSING YOUR UNIVERSITY

An excellent place to look for information about universities is the Internet: if you enter the name of the university, countless sites will pop up. Look for student nurse and nursing sites, and ask there. Current students will give you a lot of information, but they might not want to speak badly about their university. You can also search the NMC for accredited courses (www.nmc-uk.org/Approved-Programmes)

A number of factors will influence your choice of university:

- **Transport:** how will you get to class? Where will your placements be held, and how will you get to them? Is there parking?

- **Accommodation:** where will you live when you are in university, and how much will it cost?
- **The programme:** is this the kind of place you want to spend the next 3 or 4 years?
- **The size:** nurse education programmes vary in size from very small to huge – you could have 40 people or 450 people in your class.
- **Resources:** How big is the library? Is there Internet access? What is the tutor–student ratio?

You can get a list of programmes from the NMC. Find those in the area you live or where you want to live. Call those that interest you and ask them to send you information. You can also find out about them through:

- **Open days:** visiting a university, speaking to current students and finding out first hand what being a student there would be like is one of the best ways to know if you would be happy there.
- **Quality Assurance Agency (QAA):** look up the university on the QAA website (www.qaa.ac.uk). Nursing programmes are subject to audit; the QAA site will discuss the strengths and weakness of each course. You can then ask the university what it is doing to improve areas the QAA site says are a problem!
- **Other nurses and nursing students:** talk to people. Go to online nurse discussion sites, ask people at work (if you work in healthcare), ask the practice nurse at your GP's surgery, ask people in the areas you think you might want to work in as a nurse. Be prepared to hear people advise you not to go into nursing – some people are stressed and not very happy, and some people like to tease new students. Don't be put off by one bad report, either – not everyone will have the same kinds of experiences.
- **A personal visit:** if you really like somewhere, call and ask for a tour and visit on your own. Visit the student union and ask about the course. Find where students are congregating and talk to them.

If all else fails and if, after you get in, you find it is just the wrong place for you, change to a different university. After all, some trainees will find themselves moving house in the middle of their course. Changing to a different course can be complicated, but it is usually possible.

I HAVE GOT ON TO A COURSE – NOW WHAT HAPPENS?

- **Your nursing course will be academically demanding.** Make sure you have somewhere to work in relative peace and to store your library and materials. You will accumulate quite a lot of paperwork, photocopies and handouts during your course – keeping it organized from the beginning will reduce the amount of time you spend wading through huge piles of paper looking for a handout from your first module when you are at the end of your second year!

- **You will need a diary.** From the beginning of your course until the day you qualify (and into your nursing career!) you will have a varied, often hectic schedule. Although electronics are useful, back up with paper – a wall calendar is useful. A huge filofax tends to be a bit impractical (from personal experience); a small academic (18-month) diary is probably your best bet – if you use your phone, think about what would happen if you left it at home, or lost it . . . . As soon as you find out about classes, exams, assignment due dates, etc., write them down. Write down important contact details, too, for friends, hospitals, wards, placement areas, tutors, etc., as you get them.

- **Invest in a sensible, useful library.** You will need a decent nursing or medical dictionary, a drug calculations book and a study skills book. Oh, and you need both this book and the *Newly Qualified Nurses' Handbook* (did you expect me not to say that?). *The Clinical Placement*, by Levett-Jones and Bourgeois, is also really good. As far as other books, each module will tell you what is expected of you and will give a reading list. Visit the library and look at the recommended texts; once you identify those books that you find useful, it's a good idea to start your own library, beginning with a few core titles and working up to a good source of reference and specialist information. As I write this, I am faced with hundreds of books – I feel that they are old friends, waiting to help me whenever I need them to. I know them, and can easily, quickly find information. Paper is not out of date!

- **Get to know the university . . .**
  - There will usually be a bulletin board with messages about the course and a list of class sessions. Write down your class schedule as soon as you can, but check back – arrangements often change.
  - Wander around and find all the different corridors and classrooms. Get to know where the coffee shop is, where the loos are, where people relax. Nothing is worse than running late and not knowing where the classroom is.
  - Get to know everyone. It is amazing how often you will be glad that you made the effort to say 'Hello'.
  - Find the student union office and the learning resource centre/library.

If you will be living in student/university accommodation, have moved away from home for your nursing course, are an international/overseas student, are a recent school leaver or have any concerns or questions at all about life as a student, go to the student union office. They have some excellent publications (backed up by concerned and well informed staff!) to help you (see Appendix 1).

During the first few months you will be getting settled into your academic subjects and getting the mandatory training issues like lifting and handling out of the way. Many students say this is a difficult time – they want to just 'get into' nursing and get out on placements. It can be especially difficult if you have experience in healthcare. Be patient and enjoy the slow time – it soon will get so busy and hectic that the time will fly by. Plus, the information you get while waiting to 'get out there' is useful.

Courses contain two elements – the common foundation (CFP), and Branch. In CFP, you develop fundamental nursing skills common across nursing practice fields; in branch, you learn to fine tune this to your specialist area of practice.

Just a note...

Nurse education is physically, emotionally and financially stressful. Many students say that their relationships suffer during their courses, and many also say that everything went wrong in their lives while they were getting their nursing qualification. It's an intense, hectic, demanding and stressful programme. Your friends on the course will help you – they know exactly what you are going through. Among my best friends are those I met on my nursing course. Make sure as well to set aside time for friends and family who aren't on the course. You being on the course will be tough on them, too.

When the course is over, things will stabilize. When it's over, you will look back and wonder where the time went.

While you are on the course, remember: it will be terrible some days. It will have you stressed to the point of screaming. It will feel like it is never going to end. But there will also be days when you are walking on air and feel so happy you would like to dance on the ceiling. And then, before you know it, it will be over and you will be a nurse. You can do it!

FAQ

Q   I want to be a nurse but don't have the money to study . . .

A   You will never have the money. You will have more financial stability after the course than if you don't take it . . .

Q   I want to be a nurse, but I should wait . . .

A   So many HCAs I know said 'I wanted to be a nurse, but I left it . . . '. If nursing is your dream, grab it with both hands.

Q   I am disabled . . .

A   You can be disabled and be a nurse. You have to show how you can still meet the required standard, and what help you need. If you apply and are told your disability makes it unlikely you will be accepted, challenge. Speak to the Equality and Human Rights Commission in Britain or to the Equality Commission (in Northern Ireland).

Q   Should I join a Union? Isn't the Student Union enough?

A   JOIN. The Student Union will only help with academics – not with placement issues. Whether the RCN, Unison, whatever – join a union as a student. It will make a difference.

REFERENCES

Henderson, V., 1966. The Nature of Nursing. Macmillan, New York, NY

Levett-Jones, T., Bourgeois, S., 2009. The Clinical Placement: A Nursing Survival Guide. Baillière-Tindall, Edinburgh

Nursing and Midwifery Council, 2002. Code of Professional Conduct. NMC, London

Nursing and Midwifery Council, 2002. Guide for Students of Nursing and Midwifery. NMC, London

Nursing and Midwifery Council, 2007. Website information, accessed various dates throughout 2007

Royal College of Nursing, 2003. Defining Nursing. RCN, London

CONTACTS

NMC

The Nursing and Midwifery Council (NMC), 23 Portland Place, London, W1B 1PZ

Main switchboard: 020 7637 7181
Main fax: 020 7436 2924
Registrations: 020 7333 9333
Overseas applications: 020 7333 6600
Employer Confirmations: 020 7631 3200
Fitness to Practise: 020 7333 6564
Professional advice: 020 7333 6550
Press enquiries: 020 7333 6557/6558
Website: www.nmc-uk.org
E-mail: advice@nmc-uk.org

NHS information about nursing and nurse education

Provides general information about careers in nursing and midwifery, where nursing and midwifery courses are offered, how to apply for nursing and midwifery courses, funding, bursary information and other useful information.

NHS Careers, PO Box 376, Bristol, BS99 3EY

Tel: 0845 60 60 655

Fax: 0117 921 9562

Website: www.nhs.uk/careers

E-mail: advice@nhscareers.nhs.uk

Department of Health, PO Box 777, London, SE1 6XH

For publications, go to www.orderline.dh.gov.uk/ecom_dh/public/home.jsf

Specific information about nursing and nurse education in Wales, Scotland and Northern Ireland

NHS Wales Students Awards Unit, 2nd Floor Golate House, 101 St Mary Street, Cardiff, CF10 1DX/NHS Cymru Uned Dyfarniadau Myfyrwyr, 2il Lawr Ty Golate, 101 Heol Eglwys Fair, Caerdydd, CF10 1DX

Tel: 02920 261495

Fax: 02920 261499

NHS Education for Scotland, 66 Rose Street, Edinburgh, EH2 2NN

Tel: 0131 225 4365

Website: www.nes.scot.nhs.uk

E-mail: careers@nes.scot.nhs.uk

Nursing and Nurse Education in Northern Ireland

Queen's University Belfast, University Road, Belfast, BT7 1NN

Tel: 028 9024 5133

Fax: 028 9024 7895

Website: www.qub.ac.uk

Northern Ireland Practices and Educational Council (NIPEC)

Website: www.nipec.hscni.net

Relevant Organizations

Wales:

National Leadership and Innovation Agency for Healthcare (NLIAH)

Tel: 01443 233 333

Website: www.nliah.wales.nhs.uk

Scotland:

The Students Awards Agency for Scotland

   Tel: 0845 111 1711

   Website: www.saas.gov.uk

Northern Ireland:

The Department for Employment and Learning

   Tel: 028 9025 7777

   Website: www.delni.gov.uk

   E-mail: del@nics.gov.uk

2

Nursing Models

> ❝ It took me a while to get my head around all the different models, but now that I have been in a number of placements I am starting to understand how useful they are . . . They are a road map to delivering good care. ❞
>
> *Second-year student nurse*

> ❝ Nursing models are not about paper. They are not about filling out a form or completing a document – they are about the way a nurse thinks, acts and makes decisions. A nurse who relies on paperwork to care for her patient might as well pack it in and clean houses for a living, because she's no nurse. Anyone can write on a form. A nurse *thinks*. A nurse has to *think*. ❞
>
> *Nancy Roper*

In this chapter

- Nursing
- Nursing process
- Holism
- Philosophy
- Transcultural care
- Family-based care
- Nursing theory
- Framework
- Models
- Assessing yourself
- References

During your course, you will probably have at least one module that looks at nursing models and frameworks, and at the influence nursing models have on the delivery of care. This doesn't mean that this is the only place you will discuss them: nursing models and frameworks are in the background of most of the things you will do as a nurse, so of course they are in the background of most things you will do as a student! So, why do you need to know them?

- You will have modules about them
- You will need to use them for material in assessments in different modules
- You will use them on your placements
- You will take parts of them and use them to do your work as a nurse
- It makes you look brilliant when you know about them!

Here are some terms for you:

- nursing
- nursing process
- holism
- holistic care
- philosophy
- transcultural care
- nursing theory
- framework
- model/nursing model.

You will need to use these terms throughout your course and into your career.

Before you start, think for a minute:

- How do nurses know what to do?
- How do they know what to write in a patient's note?
- How do they know how to talk to people?
- How do they know what they should ask patients?
- How do they gather information and come up with an idea of what the patient needs?
- How do they make sure someone's needs are met?
- How are they certain they do the right things in the right way?

To answer all these questions, you need to think about the models, theories and frameworks that underpin the care nurses give. Although most nurses use an eclectic model (a mixed variety of bits and pieces from different models put together to make a new, individualized model), it's common that they rely more heavily on one particular model. In the UK, that model tends to be Roper; in the USA, it tends more towards Orem. The basic thing is, however, that you have to have an organized approach to patients and their care, or you won't get anything done. You need to know what you believe you should do as a nurse, what your role is, and what things you should do to provide the care your chosen group of patients needs from you.

NURSING

There is no way to define nursing succinctly, because each individual nurse comes into nursing with her own beliefs, skills and interests. There was more about the meaning of nursing in Chapter 1, but it's important to think about it again here because all the nursing models and theories stem from beliefs about the meaning of nursing. Virginia Henderson (1966) gave us one of the most common and universal descriptions of nursing:

> The unique function of the nurse is to assist the individual, sick or well, in the performance of those activities contributing to health or its recovery (or to peaceful death) that he would perform unaided if he had the necessary strength, will, or knowledge. And to do this in such a way as to help him gain independence as rapidly as possible.

Basically, Henderson says that nurses do for patients what they would do for themselves if they were able. In her discussion about nursing, Henderson identifies the different ways in which nurses assist patients, but emphasizes that the ultimate goal of nursing care is to help the individual to gain independence. Her definition tells us that nurses need to help patients find strength, to provide education to improve patients' knowledge, and to help the patients make the best decisions about their health and their care.

When the RCN started looking at definitions of nursing, it came up with six defining characteristics:

1. **A particular purpose:** the purpose of a nurse is to promote health and healing, and to care for certain groups of people based on the needs, abilities and special circumstances experienced by those people.
2. **A particular mode of intervention:** nurses do things a certain way, based on their training, knowledge and as a result of the models and theories that support their practice.
3. **A particular domain:** nurses care for people who are experiencing varying degrees of health, and the way they experience these episodes is not limited to just the body or just the mind – in order to care for the 'whole person' we must always consider the 'whole person', biologically, psychologically, socially, spiritually, culturally, economically, politically, etc.
4. **A particular focus:** nurses see the whole person, not just the one experience in which the nurse is involved. This is a key difference from the 'medical model' – a nurse doesn't see a 'diabetic', a nurse sees a person who has an illness that affects their blood sugar, which in turn means he or she needs education about diet, skin care, vision and wounds: the

nurse doesn't see 'illness', the nurse sees people that need help, support and information to live the best life possible.

5. **A particular value base:** nurses, using ethics and models, have developed a way of relating to patients and others, as people who are worthy of trust, helpful, caring and compassionate. Nurses are expected not only to exhibit these values, but to promote these values as well.

6. **A commitment to partnership:** nurses are committed to working in partnership with everyone who is involved with the patient – family, carers, other professionals; nurses realize that to work in isolation means to isolate the patient from those who can help, and this is unacceptable. The nurse isn't worried about who is in charge, but recognizes that someone must be. Nurses aren't worried about who gets the credit, but recognize that when they succeed they share the credit, and when they fail, each is accountable for her decisions and her actions.

The six defining characteristics are from the RCN document 'Defining Nursing' – the explanations are my own, but I strongly suggest you read the document. It is available in the library, online or from the RCN.

Personally, I like Henderson's definition best, although I agree the characteristics are important. I don't see them as being separate from Henderson's definition but as part of it – i.e. between the lines. What is important, however, is that you take from these definitions whatever you need to make sure you know what kind of nurse *you* need to be.

NURSING PROCESS

In the 1960s, when Virginia Henderson's definition of nursing was first published, nursing was beginning a period of dramatic change. It was growing out of being a service profession that existed only to do hygiene care and work as directed by doctors, and was becoming recognized as a profession in its own right. Nursing theorists were beginning really to look at the way nurses were thinking. One result of this was the development of the 'nursing process' – an explanation of a way of making decisions and thinking about how to deliver care.

You can use the nursing process in a number of ways: care planning, writing nurse's notes, or simply just making sure that you are using good judgement when making decisions in practice are all examples of the nursing process. There is nothing magical about it; it is simply an organized way of thinking.

There are four steps in a nursing process:

1. **Assess:** make a full assessment of the situation.
2. **Plan:** what do you want to accomplish? What goals do you have for this patient/situation?
3. **Implement:** how will you accomplish the goals?
4. **Evaluate:** how did your implementation work towards achieving the goals you set? Do you need a new plan or new method of implementation?

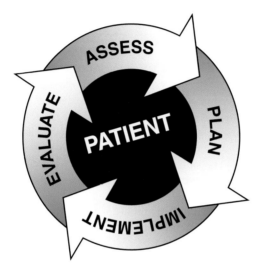

The nursing process isn't an entity by itself; it is a process through which you make decisions, record information and so on. It is also useful in more than just nursing; try it next time you pack for holiday!

HOLISM

The NMC *Code of Professional Conduct* (NMC 2002) tells you that you must respect the client as an individual. This means that you must look at all the different elements that make up your patient: the body, the mind and the spiritual self. This is the basis of holism.

Holistic care

Holism and holistic care look at the patient as a whole person, with unique and individual needs and circumstances. Holism drives the nurse to see more than just the reason patients are in care: it encourages her to look at the way patients feel, what is important to them and their families, the details of their living situation, what they believe, etc.

When discussing holism, you come across words such as 'spiritual', 'emotional', 'physiological', 'psychological' and 'cultural'. Some students might think, 'I don't know how to assess someone's psychological needs!' That's not what you have to do: try not to worry about defining these specifically – what's most important is that you remember that your patients aren't just the problem they have; they are complex people with feelings, with things on their mind, with bills to pay, a belief (or not) in good and/or the afterlife, with guilt, fear and worry, with family obligations and with expectations for themselves and others – they are just like you. Try to remember that there is more to your patient than being a patient. If you see your patients in '3D', you will give the care that best meets all their needs in a respectful and dignified way. This means remembering *never* to stereotype a patient: there is no such thing as an 'average Asian patient'; people who are Muslim will not always follow a halal diet; not all Afro-Caribbean people eat chicken and rice; and not every Asian person wants a vegetarian curry for tea. Don't assume that you know what a patient's needs are based on his or her name or appearance. How would you feel if someone thought of you as being 'average British' and fed

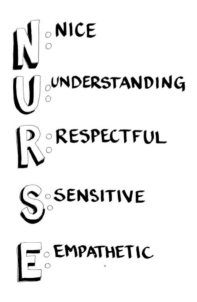

N NICE

U UNDERSTANDING

R RESPECTFUL

S SENSITIVE

E EMPATHETIC

you nothing but fish and chips? Just because someone is from a particular culture doesn't mean that he or she is a stereotype of that culture.

Making sure that you approach care in a holistic way can be difficult. That's why we use nursing models and frameworks to guide us. Nursing models, theories and frameworks are all related. Here's how they develop: an individual looks at nursing and identifies his or her philosophy. Next, that individual starts to think about nursing, about nursing care, and about the best way to meet the patient's needs. This develops into a theory. The theory then develops into a model. From the model, the individual can develop a framework – a way for the model to be applied to nursing. At some level we are all nursing theorists, because each of us develops our own beliefs, ideas and approaches to care.

The way you approach care is founded in your philosophy. Each of us has our own philosophy, even if we don't think about it actively. It can be important for your development and growth as a nurse to think about and reflect on your beliefs about nursing, the values nurses hold and the way nurses approach care.

PHILOSOPHY

A nursing philosophy is the principle a nurse, placement area or organization uses to guide the approach they have to patients, care and care delivery. Look for the philosophy in any area you are placed in, and ask yourself:

- If I were a patient, or member of staff, could I find it?
- If I were a patient, would I feel this applies to me/my care?
- Does it make sense?
- Is it too long to read? Is it too short to mean anything?
- Is it too full of buzz words to have real meaning?
- Would a staff member be able to have confidence in this?
- Would staff members say this reflects their beliefs?
- Does it make sense? Is it too idealist or too vague?
- How was it developed? Did current staff have input?
- Is it ever reviewed or updated?
- Does it reflect holism?
- Does it conflict with the *Code of Professional Conduct* in any way?

A philosophy isn't something that can simply be handed to people; it has to be something they believe in. You can learn a surprising amount about the area by looking at the philosophy: it will tell you not just what the area wants to say it believes, but about management, staff involvement and morale.

Individuals also have their own philosophy. Each of us does – we just don't often put it into words. I had a philosophy in mind when I started this book: I wanted it to be clear, direct, friendly and useful. I have my own philosophy of nursing as well. So do you. In Chapter 6, I challenge you to write it down. If you've already done that, then bravo! If not, think about it now . . . write down 'I believe that nursing is . . . ' and 'I believe that as a nurse I . . . '. This is important. You will have a clearer vision of what you are trying to achieve if you put it into words. It will help you to centre and focus yourself when you get stressed and discouraged. It will help you make better decisions if you know why you are in practice.

So, you know what you believe (your philosophy) and you know you want to address patients and their needs in a way that considers all the different aspects of their lives. You need a framework to help you, to make sure that you approach your care in an organized way and so that nothing gets left out.

TRANSCULTURAL CARE

Some models that follow in this chapter are focused not so much on washing, dressing and eating as they are on the culture of the individual. Culture is something that each of us carries, not usually consciously, but unconsciously. If I were to ask you how you are different, you might rightly say 'different from whom?', because to you all of the things about you are normal and you can't tell what aspects would be different in someone else. There are some values/behaviours you assume are shared by everyone, and some you are sure are shared by only a few.

When you look at culture, be careful not to go overboard. You can try too hard sometimes – culture isn't always what it seems to be: it isn't always what is 'written in the book'. Culture is what the person experiencing it believes it to be – so allow the patient to be your guide. Transcultural care means care *across* cultures – care that can be delivered in any culture, care that can be delivered so that people can be who they are without judgement and without bias. Instead of making your decision about what this means, allow your patients to make it for you. Ask them what their needs are, ask them what they want to eat, drink and wear. When you see your patients as they see themselves, you will have reached transcultural care in its truest form.

FAMILY-BASED CARE

Especially with children, but also whenever there is chronic or serious illness, people should be seen in the context of those who care about them and who they care about. We cannot separate people from those who are important to them, and whatever model we use, seeing someone as a part of a family is essential.

NURSING THEORY

Nursing theory is a belief or understanding about the way things are done, or should be done, in nursing. A nursing theory is an organized way of looking at nursing, nursing care and the knowledge contained in nursing. Through nursing theories, nursing practice is explored, gaps in knowledge are investigated and research is generated. This is based on a philosophy about nursing and values held by the theorist that is believed to be important. The theory is then developed, through research, investigation, audit and observation. The theory can then develop into a model – an organized approach to care based on the theory. Nursing theories are the foundation of knowledge that supports nursing practice.

There are many useful theories, but one especially useful theory is Patricia Benner's 'novice to expert'. She explains how you gain, through experience, a sense of intuition that will guide you, and in developing that experience and intuition you become an expert.

I think Benner's theory works at many levels – you become an expert new student, in time to be a novice third-year student. And just as you get really good at being an experienced student, you get pushed to the front of the 'newly qualified' queue. And on it goes. You are always developing expertise, and even the most senior nurse you know is a novice at something. It also considers expertise in different places – if you are an experienced adult nurse you are not even a novice children's nurse, but some things in children's nursing will still be familiar to you, so it will be easier for you to develop as a children's nurse than it would be for someone without nursing experience. The important thing in Benner's work is that you recognize that with experience comes intuition – an enhancement that can allow you to make decisions more quickly and that helps you think more creatively. Intuition allows you to grow and learn more easily, so you evolve more as a practitioner. Healthcare is always evolving, so nursing is always evolving, and it stands to reason that nurses are evolving too.

Benner's book *Novice to Expert* can be tough reading because it is a very theoretical book, but if you have time it's worth it.

FRAMEWORK

A nursing framework is the way a nurse organizes the care delivered to the patient. It is based on a nursing model (or a combination of models). There are different kinds of frameworks: some are meant to be on paper, some are meant to be in your head (conceptual frameworks), and some are meant to be both. An example of a paper framework is an assessment sheet that you fill in. The nursing process is an example of a framework that is in your head. Don't rely on the paper frameworks alone. It's up to you as a nurse to have a clear vision for the way you approach your care. Frameworks are built as an expression of the different models.

MODELS

A model is an example or a pattern. A nursing model is based on a philosophy that someone had about care and nursing. This developed into a theoretical approach to care and, from there, became an example and explanation of a way to apply that theory. There are many different nursing models (and theories) and many different nursing theorists. They all have some things in common, and many of them are quite similar. Models can vary based on where they were developed, what kinds of patient groups they were developed for, and the values of the people who developed them. Because all nurses are unique people, they tend to develop an eclectic model of their own – a piece of one model, a few bits from another – and this constitutes their personal approach to nursing. For this to be successful, you need experience. In the beginning, it helps to develop a strong understanding of one model: in the UK, I suggest you start with the Roper, Logan and Tierney model, only because it is used so widely.

You will find that different models use different perspectives to look at patients and their care. Some models (like those developed by Roper, Logan and Tierney) look specifically at meeting the patient's needs; other models (like Watson's) look at the nurse's interaction with the patient. Still other models will focus on the patient's environment and their adaptation within it. When looking at nursing models, try to identify the approach the theorist is taking. This will help you understand what it is the model expects you to do to care for the patient. Basing an approach to care on more than one model is being 'eclectic'.

All models involve some method of assessing patients and offering the appropriate care. A key part of the model is identifying how progress will be evaluated, so you know if what you are doing is right or if you need to do something else. Models give rise to care plans – documents that translate the care suggested into a format through which nurses can document what they are doing, and what other professionals should be asked to do. They are changed and evaluated on a daily basis as the patient's condition and abilities change.

Although all of these models can be used in any care setting, some models have evolved more out of one area of nursing than another. When the model is discussed, I will try to make it clear what specific group the model was intended for, if any.

Just as an insight into the need for models, the quote at the beginning of this chapter from Nancy Roper is a comment she made while meeting with a group of students. They were discussing all the forms and assessments they had to fill out, but when she asked them *why* they were filling out the forms, no one could come up with anything better than 'because my mentor told me to'. Nancy was passionate about promoting the value of nurses being able to think for themselves, make decisions and determine what the patient needs. She said she was disappointed that her model had turned into a paper exercise, because in making it simple it left out all the good bits – the parts of it that made sure it was holistic. Nancy died in 2004, and she is sorely missed (by most people; she had her detractors as well as admirers), but her model will live on – hopefully in its entirety as it was intended. The message here is that you need to have the basics of whatever model you choose in your *head*, using it as a road map for your nursing. If you allow someone else to write out that map for you, who knows where you will get to!

There is a multitude of models available to you; whichever you use, you must ask yourself the following:

1. Does this model allow me to gather all the information I need to make decisions about the care I need to give?
2. Does this model allow me to build a relationship with the patient?
3. Does this model allow me to meet my patients' cultural, individual and unique needs in a way that they will accept?
4. Does this model help me progress as a nurse, allowing me to do more as I know more?
5. Does this model allow me to use evidence-based practice?
6. Do I 'buy in' to this model – can I use it, believe in it and promote its use?

The Roper, Logan and Tierney model (also called Roper) is the most common model in the UK, so it will come first. The elements it contains are applicable in most of the other models, so getting comfortable with Roper will give you a good foundation no matter what you choose as a nursing destination.

Roper: the Activities of Living Model

The Roper model – developed by Roper, Logan and Tierney (2002) – asks the nurse to make an assessment of the patient based on life skills and needs, such as eating and dressing, maintaining body temperature, and being able to walk. The model was designed to look at how dependent someone is on assistance from others. One key feature many people ignore in the Roper model is that any assessment of activities of living (AL) needs to look holistically at the patient. This model is based on the Henderson theory of nursing. Although it is the most common in the UK, most nurses are familiar with only the *activities* of living, not all of the *elements*. Later in this chapter, you are asked to assess yourself based on this model.

The model asks you to consider each of the following when assessing the patient:

Activities of daily life (12 specific areas)

- Maintaining a safe environment
- Communicating
- Breathing
- Eating and drinking
- Eliminating
- Personal cleansing and dressing

- Controlling body temperature
- Mobilizing
- Working and playing
- Expressing sexuality
- Sleeping
- Dying

Lifespan: what part of life is this person experiencing, and how does that impact their independence, activities of living, etc?

- The length of time between birth and death is a person's lifespan
- Roper divides a lifespan into infancy, childhood, adolescence, adult (broken into young adult, middle years, late adulthood) and old age.

Dependence/independence continuum

- Where, on a continuum ranging from complete independence to complete dependence does the patient lie?
- What direction is the patient headed: less or more independent?
- What does the nurse need to try to do to keep them moving towards independence?
- Lifespan needs to consider – for example, how is an infant's dependence different from a person who once was independent, but who now is dependent?
- What is the greatest potential for independence, and what is the potential for dependence?
- What do you need to do to get the patient motivated towards independence or accepting of dependence?

Factors influencing activities of living

- **Biological**: nurses need to understand anatomy and physiology, in order to know about illness, so that they can promote and maintain health, prevent disease, and assess and care for those with physical illness or injury.
- **Psychological**: knowledge of psychological factors and how they affect people, including intellectual development, emotional development and psychological stressors.
- **Sociocultural**: this encompasses aspects of the person's life as social, cultural, spiritual, religious and ethical. Some of these will cause the

nurse to change the types of decisions she makes for the patient, in order to comply with the patient's beliefs and needs.

- **Environmental**: atmospheric components, including organic and inorganic particles and atmospheric pollutants; light rays; sound waves; clothing; aspects of cross-infection and hospital acquired infection; and buildings, including a person's home, nursing homes, clinics, health centres and hospitals. Under this category, the nurse needs to consider how all of these things – their presence, access and availability (wanted or otherwise) – affect the person's ability to carry out activities of living. Imagine, global warming being mentioned in a nursing model!
- **Politico-economic**: these are the factors where health is influenced by economic status, political/legal activity, industry and industrial development, and world economy, both as large global issues and how they affect an individual, such as through job availability, pensions, etc.

Individuality in living

All of the factors considered above – from lifespan to politico-economic – make a person unique, and requires the nurse to see him or her as such. Your job as a nurse is to appreciate each individual as unique, requiring you to develop an individualized approach to meeting a person's needs.

The role of the nurse

Assessment
- Collecting information from/about the person
- Reviewing the collected information
- Identifying the person's problems – both actual and potential
- Identifying the priorities among problems – your priorities and the patient's (which may differ).

Planning
- Preventing identified problems from becoming actual ones
- Solving actual problems
- Alleviating those which cannot be solved
- Helping the patient to cope positively with problems that cannot be solved or alleviated
- Preventing recurrence of a treated problem
- Helping a person to be as pain-free and comfortable as possible when death is inevitable

- Developing strategies for support and resources (such as benefits, etc.) and referring to others who can do for the patient what the nurse cannot (such as CAB, social workers, etc.), during the admission (or time when the nurse is working with the patient) and after
- Working collaboratively and cooperatively – who else needs to be involved in this person's care?
- What will this person need for discharge home (if inpatient), to stay at home, or to prevent things from getting any worse in a way that will require them to go someplace they don't want to go?
- Are there any aids, equipment or adaptations needed, either in the clinical area or at home? Who needs to be contacted to get them? What information is needed to order them?

Implementation

Implementation through:

- Listening
- Talking
- Observing
- Measuring
- Helping
- 'Not' helping
- Working with others
- Teaching
- Promoting health
- Caring
- Communicating
- Providing help or support
- Providing treatments, medications or therapies.

How are you going to help the patient reach the highest possible level of independence? How are you going to help patients make their way through whatever problems are affecting them? How are you going to help them get better, or cope with not being able to get better? Each of these steps is implementation – and starts with listening, talking, observing, helping, or 'not helping' . . . and requires more than just nursing.

Evaluation

Look at where you assessed the patient as being, and where the patient is now, and use the following:

- Observing
- Questioning

○ Examining
○ Testing
○ Measuring.

Have the implementations been effective or not effective? Has the patient benefited? Is the patient progressing towards independence? Do you need to continue the same way or change anything? Has anything happened that shouldn't have happened? Has anything that should have happened not been done?

Basically, for any part of the lifespan, Roper, Logan and Tierney can, when implemented fully, help a nurse assess and plan for the care her patient needs. The problem lies when only one part of the model is used to develop a document rather than fully assess a patient.

ACCESS Model of Transcultural Nursing

This model was developed by Doctor A. Narayanasamy, a nurse and educator, who felt that nursing students were not really given adequate information and support to understand the importance of culture and spirituality in nursing practice. ACCESS is an acronym; it outlines the way in which a nurse should approach assessment and develop the clinical environment. It is not really a nursing model; it's more of an educational model used to help student nurses develop more sensitivity to culture and spirituality. It can be used in any branch, and may be especially useful if there seems to be an obstruction between the patient and the nursing staff.

A:	Assessment of cultural aspects of life, health beliefs and health practices.
C:	Communication; look for both verbal and non-verbal communication.
C:	Cultural negotiation and Compromise; be more aware of other people's cultures and understand your patients' view of their problems – allow them to explain from their perspective.
E:	Establish respect and rapport; develop a therapeutic relationship in which there is mutual respect based on a willingness to accept the value of the patient's beliefs and culture.
S:	Sensitivity; care should be sensitive to cultural needs, to diversity and to the needs of people.
S:	Safety; people should feel that they are safe to live their life as their culture dictates, being free from others telling them their culture is invalid.

Abdellah's 21 Problems

1. To promote good hygiene and physical comfort
2. To promote optimal activity, exercise, rest and sleep
3. To promote safety through prevention of accidents, injury or other trauma and through the prevention of the spread of infection
4. To maintain good body mechanics and prevent and correct deformities

5. To facilitate the maintenance of a supply of oxygen to all body cells
6. To facilitate the maintenance of nutrition of all body cells
7. To facilitate the maintenance of elimination
8. To facilitate the maintenance of fluid and electrolyte balance
9. To recognize the physiologic responses of the body to disease conditions
10. To facilitate the maintenance of regulatory mechanisms and functions
11. To facilitate the maintenance of sensory function
12. To identify and accept positive and negative expressions, feelings, and reactions
13. To identify and accept the interrelatedness of emotions and organic illness
14. To facilitate the maintenance of effective verbal and non-verbal communication
15. To promote the development of productive interpersonal relationships
16. To facilitate progress toward achievement of personal spiritual goals
17. To create and maintain a therapeutic environment
18. To facilitate awareness of self as an individual with varying physical, emotional and developmental needs
19. To accept the optimum possible goals in light of physical and emotional limitations
20. To use community resources as an aid in resolving problems arising from illness
21. To understand the role of social problems as influencing factors in the cause of illness.

This model was developed more to help assess a student or nurse based on competency areas than to actually plan or deliver care. When I first found it, it looked too bulky, but personally I have found that picking one point and reflecting on it has been very useful and informative. This is a good example of how a model affects other models; although this might not be used on its own, it can support other models by helping nurses understand the things they need to do.

Casey's Model of Nursing

Casy, an English children's nurse, developed this model based on working in partnership. It has five concepts: child, family, health, the environment and the nurse. The principles are that the people best suited to care for a child are the child's family, but that they need help, guidance and advice to do the right things: there needs to be cooperation and partnership between the healthcare team and the family or the child will not get the best care. This is a child health model.

There is a similar model, the Nottingham model. It is very similar to Casey's, but instead of the child being the centre of the model and the family being seen as part of the therapeutic group helping the child, the family is seen as the centre.

Ecology of Health Model

This learning-disability based model, developed by Aldridge, helps the nurse to see the person with learning disabilities within a broader health context. Nurses caring for those with learning disabilities need to help their clients develop life skills that are adapted specifically to their abilities. Nurses working in this area need to develop strong health promotion and health education skills, and this model guides them to see the holistic needs of the person with learning disabilities.

Fitzpatrick's Rhythm Model

Fitzpatrick's model states that the purpose of nursing is to promote and maintain optimal health. The nurse does this through a multidisciplinary approach, using the nursing process, and in whatever the nurse does it is essential for her to be prepared to assess and meet physical, emotional, social, environmental and spiritual aspects of patients' preferences and needs.

This model has been substantial in the USA in developing the taxonomy (descriptive words) of nursing, and underpins nursing diagnosis. I wish this were a more common model here, and I would encourage any student to try to learn more about it – if for nothing more than to assess themselves as a nurse more thoroughly.

The model has four key aspects:

1. **Person:** the recognition of self and others as having unique biological, psychological, emotional, social, cultural and spiritual attitudes. All persons need honour and dignity, and strive to grow and develop as people. Many factors develop in each person's unique circumstances that will affect their health or wellness.
2. **Health:** this is the result of a person's interaction with the environment, can vary from health to illness, and changes throughout the lifespan.
3. **Wellness–illness:** nurses promote care for those across a continuum of wellness to illness, from those seeking to maintain health, to those suffering from chronic disease, to those who are dying. Nurses also must teach others to be nurses, to research nursing as a unique role, to manage and to lead, and to extend nursing knowledge and theory. Nursing centres on how nurses apply nursing theory to their efforts in maintaining, restoring or enhancing health within their place on this continuum.
4. **Metaparadigm** (i.e. things change): nursing must continue to evolve and change, because the people we care for change, the world and

society change, and all the other healthcare professionals change. If we stand still, we will become history instead of the future.

King's Model

The focus of King's model is 'on individuals whose interactions in groups within social systems influence behaviour within the systems' (King 1989). The experiences people have in their environment, and the perceptions people have about the world around them, influence their behaviour and, as a result, their health and wellness. King's model looks at personal, interpersonal and social interactions. In this model, the nurse works together with the client to determine and work towards goals and solutions (goal attainment). This is a mental health model.

Leininger: The Transcultural Nursing Model

The Leininger model emphasizes care 'focused upon differences and similarities among cultures with respect to human care, health, and illness based upon the people's cultural values, beliefs, and practices, and [using] this knowledge to provide cultural specific or culturally congruent nursing care to people' (Leininger 1978). The nursing care should bring the institution and the individual together 'in order to provide meaningful, beneficial, satisfying care that leads to health or well-being' (Leininger, p. 49). This is a general model.

Levine: Conservation Model

The nurse assesses the patient's adaptation – both personally and socially – and then supports that patient in making the necessary changes to attain and maintain 'wholeness'. The nurse helps the patient conserve energy – reducing stress and improving nutritional and physical health – by assisting him or her to adapt appropriately to the environment. This is a useful model in mental health nursing, or when the patient's lack of adaptation has made it difficult for that person to heal, such as when stress is affecting a condition like an ulcer, and so it also has applications in general nursing.

In this model, the nurse helps patients to attain wholeness, through attention to the energy they must use in order to get their needs met, the structure of the system in which their needs are met, their integrity (meaning their emotional, social and personal health), and the health of the society in which they live. Levine looks to the nurse as a guardian; one who cares for and guides the patient through a process through which they achieve health and, through this process, the nurse improves themselves and the world around them.

Neuman

In Neuman's model, the nurse is the leader of the healthcare team because the nurse's broad scope encompasses all the patient's needs. The goal is to help individuals achieve and maintain the optimum level of health possible. It encourages the nurse to identify and to help the individual identify stressors in the environment that can be controlled, helping individuals to return to a more stable, healthy state. This return to a healthy state is called 'reconstitution'. This is related to Roger's theory of energy fields. It is useful in mental health nursing.

Nightingale: Environmental Adaptation Model

Nurses must prevent the environment from contributing to impaired health and provide the foundational elements of health in order for the patient to make good use of them. Nurses must teach patients the value of these foundational elements, and encourage them to improve health. Simply put, if people eat properly, drink water, don't poison themselves, exercise properly, get enough rest and engage themselves in healthy social interaction, they will enjoy health unless the environment interferes – in which case the nurse must help them adapt to the changing environment so they can get back to taking care of themselves. A very 'Victorian' theory, but one of the first nursing theories and, in reality, it is on this theory that all nursing is based: nurses do what people would do for themselves if they were able.

Boykin and Schoenhofer: Nursing as Caring

The theory of 'nursing as caring' is a general or grand nursing theory that can be used as a framework to guide nursing practice. The theory is grounded in several key assumptions:

- Persons are caring by virtue of their humanness
- Persons live their caring moment to moment
- Persons are whole or complete in the moment
- Personhood is living life grounded in caring
- Personhood is enhanced through participating in nurturing relationships with caring others
- Nursing is both a discipline (an art based on skills and technical abilities) and a profession (a science with ethics and standards).

This model is a very different type of model; instead of looking at the patient, the patient's needs and the patient's problems, it looks at the importance of the nurse developing a caring nature, a way of looking at people with the right attitude and focus. This model guides the nurse to use respect for people and what they value as a starting point for all activities.

The developer used an image to explain the model: 'The Dance of Caring Persons'. This is an image of a circle of dancers, moving with a rhythm that connects them and organizes their movements, integrating them and making them one while also seeing them as individual people. Each person is connected, each person brings their differences, gifts and talents to the dance, and each one is 'essential in contributing to the process of living grounded in caring'. Imagine each person dressed uniquely – some with jewellery, some not, some with clanking bracelets, others quiet – and you start to get the idea.

There are two key outcomes:

- For patients, the experience of having received respectful, compassionate and competent care

- For nurses, feeling like they are 'real nurses', through promoting a respectful, caring environment.

Orem: The Self-Care Deficit Model

In this model, the nurse must identify what patients can and can't do for themselves, and then how best to help patients overcome the deficit between the two. The nurse must also identify areas where patients need education, information, support or advice to become more independent and to address any health or lifestyle problems. This is a very popular model in the USA, used extensively in general nursing.

Parent–Staff Interaction Model of Paediatric Care

This model, based on work by Linda Shields, discusses how nurses need to work with families in order to truly recognize the culture and needs of the child. It is not yet widely used; elements, however, are present in other models. So, although this seeks to heighten cultural awareness and good relationships between staff and the families of children in care situations, it is not alone in this approach. This is a child/family health model.

Peplau: The Interpersonal Relations Model

This is a common mental health nursing model.

Peplau emphasizes the development of a trusting therapeutic relationship between the nurse and the patient. The nurse and patient progress through phases as they proceed with the interpersonal process of developing this relationship. There is an emphasis on developing patients' knowledge and ability to cope, and helping them to learn the skills and gain the knowledge that they need to attain and maintain health. The role of the nurse is to identify the behaviour that interferes with health, to develop a therapeutic relationship and, through this relationship, to help patients to overcome that behaviour. There is a focus on therapeutic communication. The model states that nursing is a 'significant, therapeutic interpersonal process'.

In this model, the nurse evolves through the six roles.

Peplau's six nursing roles

These roles illustrate the dynamic character roles typical to clinical nursing:

1. Stranger role: receives the client the same way as one meets a stranger in other life situations; provides an accepting climate that builds trust.
2. Resource role: answers questions, interprets clinical treatment data; gives information.
3. Teaching role: gives instructions and provides training; involves analysis and synthesis of the learner's experience.
4. Counselling role: helps client understand and integrate the meaning of current life circumstances; provides guidance and encouragement to make changes.
5. Surrogate role: helps client clarify domains of dependence, interdependence and independence, and acts on client's behalf as advocate.
6. Active leadership: helps client assume maximum responsibility for meeting treatment goals in a mutually satisfying way.

Peplau's developmental stages of the nurse–client relationship

1. Orientation Phase: the two parties gain trust as they get to know each other relative to the environment.
2. Identification Phase: each identifies what the other wants, needs and how they must act.
3. Exploitation Phase: each gets from the other what they need; for example, the patient is in pain. The nurse wants to help, the patient wants relief. The nurse offers medication, the patient gets it, and through that they get relief and they tell the nurse the pain is gone, meaning the nurse gets satisfaction.
4. Resolution Phase: as the patient gets well, the nurse starts to withdraw the intensity of the relationship, helping the patient develop a willingness to return home. Or, if the patient will not get well, the nurse starts to prepare him or her for the next stage of life, helping the patient learn to cope with the grief he or she feels.

Rogers: Unitary Healthcare Model

The Rogers model is a complicated theory that looks at neither health nor illness, but instead focuses on patterns of energy: it looks at energy fields as the basic units of living (and non-living) things. The interaction between energy fields affects the patterns of the fields. I personally find this an interesting, but chaotic and difficult, model to follow, although it is used in mental health nursing,

Roy: Adaptive Model

In this model, the nurse is asked to see patients relative to their environment, and to assist them in adapting, in a positive way, to the circumstances in which they find themselves. Roy sees patients as people with biological, psychological and social aspects. The patients must adapt to their environment: they do this through changes in their body, in their function, in the way they see themselves and in the level of dependence they have on other people. To protect themselves, they use different coping skills. It is up to the nurse to help patients develop good coping skills, and to help them identify and resolve any negative coping skills. This is a general nursing model.

Watson: Theory of Caring

Watson outlines a number of elements in her model, but they all boil down to the following: be genuinely caring, give hope, have faith, and develop therapeutic relationships founded in non-judgemental communication that sensitively nurture patients and their families.

There are many other nursing theorists. This chapter isn't intended to teach you everything you will ever need to know about nursing models and theories, but rather to give you a head start at identifying some of the basic theories and key themes you will encounter in your course. If you want to know more, there is a lot of information on the Internet: just type the name of the model or the nursing theorist who developed it into a search engine.

One note here: nursing theory and models are living things. They are used, adapted, modified and reworked. Each one contributes to the body of knowledge and practice of nursing, and as each one follows another, it incorporates elements that have gone before. Nothing in nursing theory is a 'stand alone' concept. What that should tell you about nursing itself is that there is room for interpretation. This is exactly the reason I am encouraging you to develop your own philosophy about nursing. You don't have to choose one model to follow: find what works for you.

ASSESSING YOURSELF

By assessing yourself, you can learn a better application of the activities of living than you will learn on your own. How does being a student nurse change your activities of life? Think of the different factors – like economics – and how they impact you.

Are you the same as every other student? What makes you different? What would make a patient different?

The following self-assessment sheet can be downloaded from the Evolve website (http://evolve.elsevier.com/siviter/studentnurse/).

Activities of life

> How independent were you before you started your course?
>
> How independent are you now that your course has started?

Maintaining a safe environment

Communicating

> Do you speak differently than you did before the course started?

Breathing

Eating and Drinking

> Do you drink and eat more or less healthily now?

Eliminating

Personal cleansing and dressing

Controlling body temperature

Mobilizing

> Have your manual handling skills changed?

Working and playing

> How has work changed for you?

Expressing sexuality

Sleeping

> Bet you slept more before the course.

Dying

> Do you think of this differently now?

Summary

- Every nurse has her own philosophy of nursing.
- Holism and holistic care look at each individual as an individual with individual needs, concerns and qualities.
- There are many different nursing models: most nurses use an eclectic combination of models and frameworks in their work.
- There is no 'right' or 'wrong' model or theory; each has points that a nurse could find useful, but some are more useful than others.
- Philosophies for clinical areas should reflect the current beliefs and values of the people working there.
- Knowing any one model very well is a useful skill.
- Models should include cultural aspects as well as physical and psychological ones.
- Models can vary according to the area in which you are working, but some are universal.

REFERENCES

Abdellah, F.G., 1986. The nature of nursing science. In: Nicholl, L.H. (Ed.), Perspectives on Nursing Theory. Little Brown, Boston, MA

Aldridge, J., 2004. Learning disability nursing: a model for practice. In: Turnbull, J. (Ed.), Learning Disability Nursing. Blackwell Publishing, London, pp. 169–187

Benner, P., 2001. Novice to Expert. Prentice Hall, Upper Saddle River, NJ

Boykin, A., Schoenhofer, S.O., 2001. Nursing as Caring: A Model for Transforming Practice. Jones & Bartlett Publishers, Sudbury, MA

Casey, A., 1993. The development and use of the partnership model of nursing care. In: Glasper, E.A., Tucker, A. (Eds.), Advances in Child Health Nursing. Scutari Press, London

Henderson, V., 1966. The Nature of Nursing. Macmillan, New York, NY

King, I. M., 1989. King's general systems framework and theory. In: Riehl-Sisca, J. P. (Ed.), Conceptual Models for Nursing Practice, 3rd ed. Appleton & Lange, Norwalk, CT

Leininger, M. (Ed.), 1978. Transcultural Nursing. Wiley, New York, NY

Narayanasamy, A., The impact of empirical studies of spirituality and culture on nurse education. Journal of Clinical Nursing 15(7), 840–851

Neuman, B., Fawcett, J. (Eds.), 2002. The Neuman Systems Model, 4th ed. Prentice Hall, Upper Saddle River, NJ

Peplau, H. E., 1991. Interpersonal Relations in Nursing: A Conceptual Framework of Reference for Psychodynamic Nursing. Springer Publishing, New York, NY

Rogers, M., 1983. Science of unitary human beings: a paradigm for nursing. In: Clements, I. W., Roberts, F. B. (Eds.), Family Health: A Theoretical Approach to Nursing Care. John Wiley, New York, NY

Roper, N., Logan, W., Tierney, A., 2002. The Elements of Nursing, 4th ed. Churchill Livingstone, Edinburgh

Watson, J., 1999. Postmodern Nursing and Beyond. Churchill Livingstone, Edinburgh

Further Reading

Alsop-Shields, L The parent–staff interaction model of pediatric care. Journal of Pediatric Nursing 17(6): 442–449

Bulfin S, Mitchell GJ 2005 Nursing as caring theory: living care in practice. Nursing Science Quarterly 18(4): 313–319

Halterman TD, Dycus DK, McClure EA et al 1998. Nursing Theorists and their Work, 4th edn. Mosby, St Louis, MO

Heather A, Roy C 1999 The Roy Adaptation Model, 2nd edn. Prentice Hall, Upper Saddle River, NJ

Kozier B, Erb G, Blais K et al 1998 Fundamentals of Nursing: Concepts, Process, and Practice, 5th edn. Addison Wesley Longman, Menlo Park, CA

Nursing and Midwifery Council 2002 Code of Professional Conduct. NMC, London

Pressler JL 1996. Fitzpatrick's rhythm model. In Fitzpatrick JJ, Whall AL (eds) Conceptual Models of Nursing: Analysis and Application, 3rd edn. Appleton & Lange, Stamford, CT, pp. 305–329

Riehl-Sisca J (ed) 1989 Conceptual Models For Nursing Practice, 3rd edn. Appleton & Lange, Norwalk, CT

Smith F 1995 Children's Nursing in Practice: The Nottingham Model. Oxford: Blackwell Science

3

Academic Work

'I haven't had to write a paper since school!
I had to take the access course and although it really gave me a lot, I was still really intimidated by the kinds of assignments I had to do in the nursing course. I worked really hard on them, and did well – a lot better than I thought I would do. I've just finished my course and I'm starting my community nurse job. My advice to a new student? Don't put things off, and get support from your tutors. You'll do just fine.'

Jane (who was 34 when she started her nursing course)

In this chapter

- Referencing
- Plagiarism
- Writing an assignment
- Confidentiality and privacy
- Basic IT skills
- References
- Assignment information worksheet

This will be a dull, boring chapter. It is filled with little details that, although useful, are not very inspiring. But I can promise you that they will help you get better grades. Trust me.

First, please keep in mind that the topic of this chapter is 'academic work'. I am introducing a couple of key concepts first, but this is because these concepts are so fundamental. If you don't reference properly, or if you plagiarize, then no matter how well the paper is written it won't matter because you will fail.

In any circumstance where the advice I give you or the advice you find conflicts with the university, unless you can prove absolutely that the university is *wrong* then go with what the university staff tell you . . . they are assessing you and they know what they want as proof from you. It's small consolation to be right if the university doesn't agree!

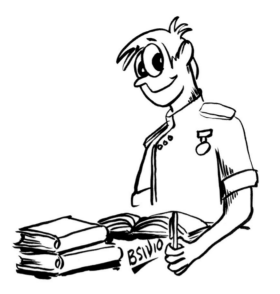

REFERENCING

An excellent paper, which would have been worthy of an A if not so poorly referenced.

Feedback on a paper graded 'C'

Referencing properly does a number of things for your work. It shows:

- how widely you have read
- how critically you have looked at ideas and concepts
- that you can follow directions
- that you give credit properly to others for their ideas and work.

Students often find that poor referencing is an easy way to lose grades. You will work really hard, finding sources, making them work together . . . then lose a mark because references weren't written out just the way the university wants them! Some hints:

- You will find yourself using the same sources over and over in many different modules, so keep your reference lists from all your assignments. Make sure your references are accurate and complete.
- Get – and keep – a copy of your university's referencing guidelines.
- Whenever possible, use references your instructor refers to in lectures and gives you in handouts. When they use them in their lectures, they

are telling you that they value them and the information in them. How much more of a hint could that be? One thing though – they probably know those references inside out.

What doesn't need to be referenced?

There are some things that don't need to be referenced:

- common knowledge (e.g. grass is green)
- undisputed facts (e.g. David Beckham was captain of the England team that played in the 2002 world cup, or Frank Skinner is a Baggies fan).

What does need to be referenced?

Things that *do* need to be referenced are:

- a quote, or ideas summarized or paraphrased and taken from another text or source, such as an Internet page.
- statistics, figures, diagrams or other visuals taken from any other work. Those generated as a result of the work you have done yourself in your paper don't need to be referenced.
- things that could be challenged (e.g. 'inflation decreased last year'). A reference gives proof that your information is accurately reported. (Don't take it for granted that just because it was published it is correct. A reference tells the reader you are being accurate: your arguments in the paper tell them you are right!)

Your university or nursing programme will tell you about the type of referencing it expects you to use. If you need more information, you can check on the Internet by searching for 'how to reference' or for the specific reference style (e.g. 'Harvard referencing') on a search engine. You can also get a study guide. There is a list of suggested sources in the Useful Books, Journals and Other Resources section at the end of this book.

PLAGIARISM

Due to cheating by plagiarism, the university has no choice but to exclude you from your course. This action will be reported to the Student Grants Unit and to [Nursing and Midwifery Council] . . . .

From a letter to a student who submitted
an essay purchased on the Internet

Your credibility is on the line when you write a paper. You must make sure you are being fair and honest – dishonesty can cost you, not just in grades, but possibly also your place in your course, and your nursing career.

The word 'plagiarism' comes from the Latin word '*plagium*', which means 'kidnapper'.

(Pickett et al. 2000)

If I had made the above statement without a citation, you might say 'How does she know that?' You would have a right to ask! Finding out I don't speak Latin, you would wonder:

- is that the truth or did she just make it up?
- did she look it up, but isn't saying she did because she wants me to think she knows a lot?
- was she too lazy to write down where it came from?

Is that how you want your markers to be looking at your work and exams? I expect you would rather let them know that you are intelligent and that you are fair and honest; plagiarism is theft. In most universities, plagiarism will get you thrown off the course on the first occurrence; it is an extremely serious academic offence. No matter how stressed you are, no matter how appealing 'www.buy-your-assignment-here.com' looks, it's not worth the risk to take a temporarily appealing, but completely dishonest and unprofessional, shortcut. It's **cheating**. People who cheat are not trustworthy. The Code of Conduct says nurses should always be trustworthy. Catch my drift?

Many people who plagiarize do it unintentionally:

- They might think that they only need to cite something if they quote it directly
- They might lose information about a source and include the information anyway (but is that titbit of information worth failing your entire assignment or exam for?)
- They might have worked closely with another student and shared information and ideas (you must show that you did your work independently!).

In any case, there will be no excuse if you are found to have plagiarized something. I represented a student recently at a disciplinary hearing. She had worked with her university roommate on a particularly difficult paper; only her roommate had gone for a tutorial, and had afterwards shared her notes with her friend who had missed the class. The tutor, who read both papers, noticed right away that they were similar: the same references, the same concepts and the same topic. Although the students openly admitted they had worked together, each claimed that she had written her own paper. The university disagreed, and both students failed the module. They were given written warnings and had to repeat the assessment. What seemed like a good work-saver cost them the chance for a first class honours degree; it could have cost them their careers in nursing.

If you are unsure of what needs to be cited and what doesn't, ask your tutor or someone in your university's academic resource centre or library. Personally, I have cited things that I didn't really need to just to give extra weight to my argument and to be certain that there was no chance I could be accused of cheating.

Once you have the right question, you need to frame the paper in an outline: this is a skeleton on which you hang the paper to give it form and structure.

WRITING AN ASSIGNMENT

> I keep telling myself, get it done, get it done – but I always find myself in a panic the weekend before it is due trying to write a huge assignment. This is hell! Why do I keep doing this to myself?
>
> *Excerpt from a student nurse's reflective diary*

In my experience, most students fail assignments because of one of three things:

1. They submit a beautifully written, well thought-out essay that unfortunately doesn't answer the question the assignment brief asked!
2. They have rushed to do the assignment at the last minute and haven't had time to proofread it and polish it up.
3. They don't know how to structure an assignment.

When you get your initial module guide for a given module, it will usually include an assignment brief, although sometimes the assignment brief will come later.

An assignment brief should include:

- the title of the assignment
- a list of suggested topics (usually)
- a description of the purpose of the paper
- the word limit
- the deadline and submission information
- learning outcomes
- a marking matrix (sometimes, but not always).

Make sure you understand the question. I know a nursing student who wrote an assignment on incontinence for a module called 'Care of the chronically ill'. She had beautiful graphs and charts, discussed different care products, wrote about an incontinence assessment, outlined the complications of incontinence and the causes of incontinence, looked at the patient holistically, had good references and presented the assignment flawlessly. She failed. The problem? The assignment brief listed 'will discuss the nursing management of a group of patients with this need' and 'will reflect upon the work of the nursing team in improving patient outcomes'. Her paper talked a lot about the problem, but didn't touch on those learning outcomes. When you finish your paper, read it through and check off elements that meet the learning outcomes. Make sure you have them all covered.

Some modules may give you a marking matrix. This should tell you all the elements that are expected to be included in the assignment, and how heavily they will be weighted.

You should also consider the level at which you are doing the assignment. Common foundation work is usually assessed at a lower standard than branch, and work at bachelor's degree is higher than work at diploma level. The higher the academic level, the more you will be expected to challenge and be critical (questioning) about what you see and learn.

Answering the question

The first part of every paper is the question: this is the topic you will discuss, investigate, examine, contrast and compare until you are so sick of it that you never want to look at that topic again. It is the thing that you take through the paper and come out with at the end, neatly wrapped and ready for consumption by your tutor.

Getting the topic right is the only way to pass, and it's not as easy as it may sound. There are two ways to get the right topic:

1. It is assigned to you
2. You choose it.

If it's assigned to you, it's pretty easy really. You just do what it tells you. But sometimes there is a topic you are really interested in that isn't one of the suggested topics. You may want to ask your marker if you can do this topic instead of one of those listed. There are pros and cons for doing this.

Pros:

– Doing a unique topic can sometimes show you are innovative and creative
– A marker who has just read 60 essays on one topic might be relieved to find that essay 61 is unique
– It's always more fun to do something that you are interested in.

Cons:

– The marker may be looking for proof that you have achieved certain outcomes and your topic might not show the right kind of proof
– The marker may have a bias towards a particular perspective or approach to topics
– The marker may feel that you haven't followed the assignment brief
– Something that was interesting might fade a bit after writing a comprehensive assignment about it.

How do you get around the cons? First, always discuss the choice of topics with the tutor. If you negotiate for an original topic, get it in writing!

The information you are given in class will also guide you to what is expected from the assignment. If you are being given information about certain models, theories or concepts, the marker will probably expect to see them in your assignment.

There are other hints as well. For example, if the learning outcomes are:

- student can express how psychological and physical health are interrelated
- student can appreciate how culture affects care decisions,

then will a paper on choice of diet do you any good? Probably, but you have to frame it properly. What would you talk about: how the dietician was involved, or why people choose the food they do?

One of the best ways to be sure you are answering the right question in the right way is to ask for a tutorial, provided tutorials are available. Tutors may not appreciate hundreds of requests for individual tutorials, but, personally, if a tutor is going to mark your paper, I think you have a right to talk to them individually about the paper. Especially if you aren't sure what you need to do to give *them* the proof they need to know that *you* know what you are talking about. I love helping students prepare for a paper I've asked them to do – it's so much easier than hashing my way through a poorly written paper.

Always book an appointment for tutorial help. Dropping in might seem easier, but neither you nor the tutor is really ready and it won't be the best use of anyone's time. Don't wait – book your tutorial early to make sure you get one. If the module tutor isn't available, go to your personal tutor. But, no matter who you go to, if the tutor is going to give up valuable time to help you, you should be respectful and not waste a moment of that time. Show up on time, ask the tutor how much time you have, and don't chit-chat: get to the point and ask what you need to ask. It won't do you any good to have a tutorial before you have an idea of what you will be writing about. Bring a basic outline with you and always write down ideas. As soon as you walk out of the office, you will forget most of what was said – write it down! If you go in with a number of different ideas, get your tutor's feedback on what he or she likes. When you qualify, you can write whatever you want. When you are a student, like it or not, the goal is to give back to your tutors what they want. This is because they have to prove you met the criteria to pass the course, and that's what's most important to you too, isn't it?

Structuring your assignment

Every assignment you write should have four main parts:

1. **The introduction:** you use this section to tell the reader what is coming. Using your module guide, assignment guide and marking matrix, map out what you are going to talk about. Try to have a logical flow from one area of discussion to another.

2. **The body:** in this part, you follow the pattern set in the introduction. Link paragraphs logically, and watch your continuity.
3. **The conclusion:** this is where you summarize everything else, and reaffirm that you have covered what you promised to cover.
4. **The reference list:** the sources you cited in the paper.

A mistake many students make is not organizing their information properly. Don't worry if you aren't a great writer – having good flow and good writing styles will get you good grades, but you don't need to be Charlotte Brontë to pass. In a minute I will give you some ideas about how to outline your paper. A good outline will make your paper easier to write.

A mistake many students make is writing in the wrong 'voice'. Some of the reference papers you read as background will be in an academic style, which means that instead of saying (for example) 'I agree . . . ', the author must say 'this student agrees . . . ' or 'the author agrees . . . '. Informal writing or narrative writing allows the author to 'speak' in first tense. This book is written in narrative style – as though I am talking to you. Make sure you know what 'voice' your tutor wants for the paper. Usually, reflections can be done in a narrative voice, but everything else needs to be in academic voice.

You are now aware of the right voice, and you are sure you have the right topic; next you need to prepare a 'skeleton' called an outline. You can use this to organize your paper, to structure it and make sure it has a clear, orderly and complete presentation.

Let's use the 'choice of diet' idea. My assignment brief says I need to write a paper of 1500 words that will discuss how the choices a patient is given in the clinical area affect their health, and how their health is not only physical; and highlight how the nurse needs to promote good health. Looking at the learning outcomes, I know I have to include something about physical and psychological health, and I need to look at how culture affects decisions. How culture affects decisions? . . . Is that my decision as the nurse or the patient's decision? I think I will add that in the paper. Now, I need to prepare that outline.

Introduction

This part is the body of my paper:

2 Case study: my patient
    2.1 Mention confidentiality
    2.2 Give an outline of my patient's general health
    2.3 Talk about culture
3 Psychological and physiological aspects of diet
    3.1 Talk about culture and diet
    3.2 Talk about how choices differ from availability

4   The nurse's role in promoting diet and health choices
   4.1   Talk about reflection and why the nurse has to recognize her own culture and its influence
   4.2   Talk about health promotion
5   Summary (this is the last part of the body of my paper)
6   Conclusion
7   References.

If I bring this to my tutor, she might like it or might not. I will make notes about what she says, and then ask her to sign off my notes so I know I have evidence that she told me to write it that way. She might say I shouldn't use a case study.

Just a thought here – if I choose a real patient to use, do I need to ask his permission? If I change his name, does he need to know he is in my paper? Yes, he does – you need to ask the patient if you can study him for a paper. Most patients will say yes, but that doesn't mean you can get away without asking.

Back to the outline: as I gather information, I can put 4.1 or 2.1 on it, depending on where it fits in the outline, to help me organize. I can make sure that every time I talk about culture and diet, it's in the same place so I don't skip around.

When I write the paper, I can then allocate the number of words I have to each section, to help me keep it balanced.

I will schedule at least two more tutorials – the very first, I made sure I had the right topic. The next, I make sure that I am moving in the right direction – this is about 3–4 weeks before the paper is due. The final tutorial, if everything has basically been going well, is 2 weeks before the paper is due. At this point, the paper should be very nearly written and I can go over it in depth with my tutor. I will watch her body language and facial expressions, and I will take good notes, adding in and changing anything she tells me.

Never send your paper to anyone other than a course or personal tutor who has specifically requested it for review and help:

- Tutors won't read papers they haven't requested
- Colleagues might nick it and submit it as their own.

Timing it right

You need to plan a time frame for your paper. Use your diary or a calendar to plan deadlines for the different stages of your assignment. The last page of this chapter is a photocopiable outline for each paper; the same form is also downloadable from the Evolve website for this book (http://evolve.elsevier.com/siviter/studentnurse/).

My suggestion is that you:

- write in your diary the date the paper is due, then back-track 1 week and write it in again as due. Try to get it done by the earlier date.
- make deadlines for yourself: when the first draft will be done, when your tutorial will be, etc. Stick to them.
- save copies of all your work on *two* separate disks or external drives, as well as on your computer, in case one copy is corrupted or lost. Don't save anything on a university or shared computer. One way to back-up is to e-mail yourself your assignment!

Preparing for your assignment

There is a lot you must do to prepare for your academic assignment:

- **Know what is expected of you:** what the question is that the assign-ment is answering, and the format expected of the completed work.
- **Research your sources:**
  Have a referencing guide to make sure your references are done properly. Have a study guide book to help you map out, plan and complete your assignments.
- **Leave enough time to do your work.** Although assignments done at the last minute can be successful, they are hell on your spirit, your sense of humour and the bags under your eyes. Get it done sooner and be lounging about with a pint in the student union bar while your friends are panicking.

If you leave it until the night before to type up your assignment, I can guarantee that some of the following will happen:

- Your computer will crash, eating all but 8 words of your 3000-word assignment on wound care, just as a burglar breaks into your house and steals your only back-up copy.
- You will run out of paper, ink, electricity and/or brain cells.
- You will oversleep and pass the assignment in 4 minutes after the deadline.
- Your sister will break up with her fiancé and spend all evening sitting in your room, eating chocolate-chunk ice cream and crying all over you.
- You will meet the perfect partner and have to choose between writing about the joys of leg ulcer care or jetting off to a holiday in Crete.
- Your two best friends from the course will have done the same thing and be on the phone to you in a panic begging to work together.
- Your friend who did her work early will be gloating at you from her seat in the student union bar.

When you get your assignment back . . .

- Look at the feedback and look through the paper for any notes or comments. Use the feedback to guide the way you write other papers. If you disagree strongly with any of the comments, bring them to the marker's attention.

- Keep the assignment. It has information in it that has already been critiqued. It could be useful for other work!

If you do particularly poorly on an assignment, make an appointment to speak to the tutor. Ask to review the marked copy of the paper. Make a note of the points raised so you can do better next time.

If you struggle to write assignments, get a tutorial from your university's student support services, ask the student union if it has workshops on assignment writing, ask another student for help, approach a tutor and ask for help, or look at one of the books listed in the Useful Books, Journals and Other Resources section at the end of this book.

Some final points: don't leave your assignments lying around; don't leave them on the 'generic desktop' of university computers; don't give them to other people (who may copy them). You are working really hard; don't let someone steal your hard work. If two people hand in similar assignments, it will be noticed and both parties could be called before a Cheating Board. Make your life simple: keep your assignments to yourself.

CONFIDENTIALITY AND PRIVACY

I was in the lift talking about my patient to my friend on the course. I didn't say his name or anything, so I thought it was OK. Later, a lady who had been in the lift with us came to visit my patient. The look on the visitor's face said it all when she saw me. I felt dreadful.

First-year nursing student

As a student nurse, and continuing as a nurse, you will have access to sensitive and personal information about patients and their families. They may be your friends, your neighbours, well-known people, or people who are in particularly delicate circumstances. You have an obligation to keep that information private. If you fail to maintain confidentiality, your patients could suffer and so will your grades. You could even find yourself excluded from the course.

Always blank out the name of hospitals and wards on documents you put into any written assignment – you should never refer to any trust or facility by name. Instead of 'Clipper one, the Gynaecology Ward at Smythfields NHS

Trust', you should put 'on a gynaecology ward of a local trust'. Community hospitals serve people who live and work locally. It wouldn't be hard for someone to (correctly or incorrectly) work out that their 42-year-old neighbour who was recently in the hospital could be the 42-year-old man suffering from alcohol withdrawal who was discussed in your paper, especially if he lives in the same area as the hospital you mentioned. Again, it's not just ethics at risk here, it's your grades. You will lose marks if you don't handle information sensitively and professionally.

You also have to be careful about the manner in which you refer to patients. Being judgemental makes you look unprofessional. How would you feel about each of the following statements?

> The patient was abusive and rude, and staff had to force him to wash. His smell offended other patients, probably because he slept rough. He was a filthy mess but his skin was OK.

and

> The patient had a long history of alcoholism and had been homeless for some time. He appeared distressed and upset. His hygiene was poor, so staff assisted him in bathing. Skin and nutritional assessments were done.

These two paragraphs say the same thing about the patient – but different things about the nurses who wrote them. Being unprofessional will cost you marks. It also shows your lack of fitness to be a nurse.

There are some important points that you must remember about patient privacy and written assignments:

- You must ask permission from patients if you are using them as a case study or will be referring to them in your paper or documentation for your university.
- You must change identifying information about them so no one can tell who they are by your description.
- Note in your paper that you are using a pseudonym (cite it – show you know the rules!).
- Never identify the ward, trust or area in which you cared for the patient except in general terms.
- You must be professional in your descriptions and observations, never judgemental or biased.

Also, never refer to classmates or work colleagues by name in your papers. It is an issue of privacy for them, too. How would you feel if one of your classmates referred to you by name? Always keep details of everyone – the trust, the staff, the patients – confidential.

BASIC IT SKILLS

Which are you?

A. I remember when calculators first came out. They were big, bulky and expensive. I still use a slide rule. I hated technology then and I hate it now. I write my assignments in pencil.

B. I have a computer. I don't know what kind, but it has Office on it.

C. My computer is a Pentium 26z with 4096 gig of RAM, a CD-RW, a DVD player, surround-sound speakers, a built-in microwave, seating for 10 and a panoramic webview of the Edgbaston cricket ground. Oh, and the voice-activated software has been trained to call in my pizza order by remote control.

Whichever you are, you will probably need to use a computer during your nurse education:

- to write assignments
- to research information on the Internet and in the library
- to use study materials found on CD/DVD
- to play games when you are so stressed you want to run away from home
- to e-mail family and friends who are not on your course to tell them that, although they haven't seen or heard from you in weeks, you are still alive, just working on an assignment
- on placements, for patient details and records.

Most universities have tutorials on computer usage. If you are:

- Person A: go; don't be afraid. Computers are (usually) pretty easy to use and, with the right support, you will be able to build skills and confidence
- Person B: go; you will build confidence and learn easier ways to do things you already know how to do
- Person C: go; you will be a support to your friends and classmates. Don't be tempted to do all their work online for them – you won't have time to get your own done if your friends all look to you as the resident net guru.

If your university or nursing programme does *not* have IT tutorials, find out why! It should be preparing you to use computers as part of your eventual work as a nurse. Look into getting the European Computer Driving Licence (ECDL) – it is easy, can be free, and gives you all the skills you need. In this day and age, you cannot afford to be computer shy. Although many people read-ing this may think, 'Hey, everyone knows computers!', remember that there are generations of people still young enough to be in nurse education who are old enough to remember when a hard drive was the bank holiday journey to Devon, completed in the pouring rain accompanied by a 5-hour chorus of 'are we there yet?'. Be patient with us!

If you don't have a computer or Internet access, your university should have a computer room with access. Remember to take your disks or USB pen to save information on, and don't forget that in peak times (when assignments are due) it could be very difficult to access a computer. Plan ahead.

Some universities have a loan service for laptops; if so they will go quickly, so look into it right away.

Floppies have fallen out of use: get yourself re-writable disks, but for real ease get as large a USB pen as you can afford, with security features to prevent theft of your work – and make sure it has your name on it! Put a file called 'IF THIS IS FOUND' as a document, on the 'insecure' part of the pen. And don't forget to run virus scanning on anything you use to connect to the Internet or a public computer.

There are some great books that can help you with using different com-puter programs – I love the . . . *For Dummies* books. Even as an experienced computer user, I find them useful.

Other resources can be found in your library. Useful search engines, such as Ovid and the British Nursing Index (BNI), catalogue periodicals. Some on-line resources and databases that you can access from home or university require you to have an 'Athens' password. They are free to students who have registered through their university. Speak to the librarian or IT helpdesk to find out how to get access to Ovid, the BNI and CINAHL, and how to get an Athens password.

See if there is information on 'how to search'. It may sound simple, but knowing how to search properly is a very valuable skill. Some learning resource centres run short courses to help you gain confidence in searching. It's a good investment. Although there is a little about literature searches in Chapter 9, it is too vast a skill for me to teach you here. Your learning resource centre/university library is the best place to start if you need to learn to search for sources and information. A short list of resource books appears in the Useful Books, Journals and Other Resources section at the end of this book.

REFERENCES

Pickett, J., 2000. The American Heritage Dictionary of the English Language, 4th ed. Houghton Mifflin, Boston, MA

Assignment information worksheet (you can download a copy from the Evolve website http://evolve.elsevier.com/siviter/studentnurse/)

Submission check list:

☐ Spelling checked

☐ References double checked

☐ Correct voice and tense used throughout

☐ Counted words correct

☐ Went over advice from all tutorials

☐ Reference list properly formatted

☐ Printing left no marks or smudges

☐ Have the right folder to submit it in

☐ All pages except first have page numbers

☐ Paper is formatted according to University guidance

☐ Have cover sheet with module name, number and assignment name

☐ Have hidden all identifying marks on any documents included

☐ Have attested to patient confidentiality

☐ Have used and referenced Code of Professional Conduct

☐ Paper clearly meets the learning outcomes and goals from module

Module Number: **Module Leader:**   **Voice:**

Module Name: Number of Words: Due Date:

Topic Chosen: _____ Dates due: Outline: _____
_____ First draft: _____
_____ Second draft if needed: _____
_____ Final draft: _____
_____ Paper completed by: _____

Tutorials: list date and overview of items discussed

First Tutorial Date	Second Tutorial Date	Final Tutorial Date
☐ Topic Chosen	☐ Outline Done	☐ Final Draft
Date:	Date:	Date:
Date Submitted:	Date Returned:	Grade Received:

What I learned that I need to apply to other papers

© **Elsevier Ltd 2013**

Clinical Placements

4

> ❝On my first placement, I was walking through the ward and I heard a patient cry out 'Nurse! Nurse!' Suddenly, I realized she meant ME! – I was the nurse! ❞
>
> *Student nurse reflective diary*

> ❝When I was a student, I used to throw myself together and pray I made it in on time – then after I qualified, I saw a student who looked like I must have done – a bit of a mess, actually, trousers wrinkled, shoes that had the wrong heel for manual handling ... and not prepared at all. I thought 'How am I going to pass her?' and then remember those nurses who passed me. The same curse that gets you kids like the child you were works with student nurses I think! If I could do it all over, I would be on time more often! ❞
>
> *New nurse*

In this chapter

- Nurse education changes in the late twentieth century
- The Peach Report
- Making a difference
- The branches of nursing
- Clinical placements
- Supernumerary status
- Becoming a nurse one placement at a time
- Mentorship
- Other people who help you learn
- References
- Clinical placement checklist

🔍 Just a note...

When I say 'ward', I mean any area in which you have a placement.

There have been enormous changes in the NHS over the past 20 years. This chapter concentrates on those that affect nurse education, while Chapter 1 outlined some of the more recent changes (through the Agenda for Change) on the grading, promotion and payment of nurses.

This history will give you a background as to why nurse education is configured the way it is. Many of you will become mentors yourselves, and it's best to learn from the mistakes and actions of the past. Knowing about how nurse education moved into universities is part of that past that has made us who we are.

NURSE EDUCATION CHANGES IN THE LATE TWENTIETH CENTURY

Nurse education has changed dramatically since the 1980s. Once, nursing students were employed by hospitals as apprentices. They were educated in the hospital; they worked on and staffed the wards. They learned everything through experience. These students often had the same responsibilities and demands placed on them as the staff nurses. It would not have been uncommon to go onto a ward and find a senior student supervising junior students, with no sign of a staff nurse anywhere.

However, it was decided that nurse education had to become more academically based. Nurses had good skills, but not enough theory or evidence to help them progress as things changed. In 1989/1990, Project 2000 was introduced. This took what had formerly been called 'pupil' or 'apprentice' nurses and made them into students – and not just in name; it took the base for training nurses out of the clinical areas and moved it to universities.

There were some radical changes: nursing students would now be supernumerary, where previously they were used to help staff clinical areas. They would receive an education to prepare them both academically and clinically. They would have the benefits and support that come with being a full-time student.

Although this change was heralded by many as the most significant ever to have occurred in nurse education, some people were very worried that it was the death knell for competent clinical practice. In 1999, the Department of Health (DH) admitted that, in many ways, Project 2000 was not meeting the needs of the modern NHS. In part, this finding was based on the Peach Report.

THE PEACH REPORT

The Peach Report – also called *Fitness for Practice* (UKCC 1999) – looked at the nature of nurse education and made recommendations to 'prepare a way forward for pre-registration nursing and midwifery education that enable fitness for practice based on health care need' (UKCC 1999, p. 2). The recommendations provided guidance for making nursing students into nurses who were fit for practice and fit for purpose.

Recommendation 10 in the Peach Report states that 'consistent clinical supervision in a supportive learning environment during all practice placements is necessary' (p. 37), and a number of recommendations suggest that higher education institutes and service providers (trusts, placement areas, etc.) should work together to provide the best education for students (UKCC 1999).

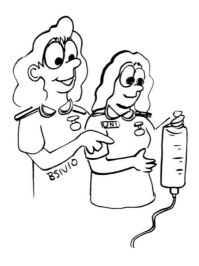

MAKING A DIFFERENCE

Following the Peach Report, the DH published *Making a Difference* (DH 1999). This set out a number of priorities for nurse education: it should be more flexible, modern and responsive, and something that fits with modern life. Students needed the protection of being students, but they also needed to be fit for nursing at the end of the course! Despite these changes, one thing that did not change was the branch structure.

When it became clear that nursing education was still not providing us with the right kinds of nurses (and not providing nurses with the right development), we recognized that nursing needed a different approach. So we put out a huge consultation about pre-registration nurse education – and the NMC developed a framework for universities on how they would deliver education to prepare knowing and skilled but also critically thinking and caring nurses. Parity between the countries in the UK was essential (so all-degree became the norm), and finances needed to be addressed. Students would have less financial support, but more access to a degree than ever before. Nurse education would enter the twenty-first century, starting in 2013. This work was done by the Professional Practice and Registration Committee, which I joined specifically so I could be there to speak for students, and their need to get a good education that served as a strong foundation for professional practice. Oh, and to make sure disabled students got reasonable adjustments – I wanted to get that in there too.

THE BRANCHES OF NURSING

The Peach Report (UKCC 1999) also recommended a review of the current branch structure of nurse education. As discussed in Chapter 1, there are currently four branches in pre-registration nurse education: adult nurse, children's nurse, mental health nurse and learning disability nurse. Whereas Peach suggested that the branches needed to be reviewed, many other people have suggested that a return to 'generalist' education is needed; however, the pre-reg review decided to look at middle ground – we would keep the branches, but students would not only have more exposure to other branches, but would also be asked to think about how care connected through the fields of practice.

The UK is the only country in the world to separate nurse education into these four branches, and this makes it difficult for nurses qualified in a branch other than adult nursing to register and work in other countries. However, nurses in the branches other than adult nursing feel that they have been specially prepared to care for vulnerable specialized patients. This will be an ongoing issue.

You will have placements in your own area of nursing. In addition, you will probably have a placement in three of the following areas (not including your own branch) to familiarize you with the different branches: you will also be asked to think about each person, family and community as holistically as possible. The branches are:

- child health
- learning disability
- mental health nursing
- maternal health (midwifery isn't a branch, but it is a specialist area of practice)
- adult nursing.

Placements can be in a number of different areas and formats, including:

- in a public-sector hospital, care home, GP practice or other facility
- in a private-sector hospital, care home or other facility

- in a school, nursery or with school nurse
- in the community with health visitors or district nurses
- independently arranged (electives) in which students find the area in which they wish to take a placement
- private study (usually done with a workbook or to produce a piece of academic work that reviews a clinical area)
- overseas placements and electives. These can be very complicated to arrange, as well as expensive, so if you are interested in going to another country for a placement you need to speak to your personal tutor and the allocations department and look for funding as soon as possible. If you wait, the placement might not be possible. The Royal College of Nursing has written some helpful guidance on overseas placements for nursing students. Don't set your heart on an overseas placement; they are almost impossible to arrange or to get approved.

Because of the increasing number of nursing students, it can be very difficult for the university to place all the students within a certain geographical area. This means that more and more students are finding that they need to travel quite long distances to their placements, or that they are being given an alternative placement such as private study, although the NMC is tightening its permission on such non-clinical placements. It also means that mentors and staff nurses in clinical areas are often stretched to provide the supervision and support that student nurses need.

So, what does this mean to you on placement?

CLINICAL PLACEMENTS

Your placements will take place in different areas and usually in different trusts. You will be relying on staff nurses and other staff members (such as physiotherapists, doctors, etc.) to help meet your learning outcomes and gain the experience you need to become a qualified nurse.

A few things to remember:

- **Patients have the right to say no to having a student care for them.** When you introduce yourself, tell patients you are a student and make sure you have their permission. Don't assume.
- **You have more to prove than any other member of staff.** Dress and look the part of an eager and well-prepared student. Clean, appropriate uniform and appearance will score you immeasurable points with staff and patients alike. Staff will be looking at you critically – don't give them any cause to doubt you.
- **Nail varnish and make-up.** These can be vectors for infection (i.e. carry infective material that can get into a patient's wounds), and cologne, perfume and make-up can all be allergens. People with allergies and

breathing difficulties can be made very ill by exposure to these; don't use them on placements.

- **Rings, bracelets and long fingernails.** These can scratch patients and can be vectors for infection. Don't wear them. You might lose them or ruin them anyway.

- **If your hair is long, tie it back.** This is as much for your safety as it is for cleanliness.

- **Necklaces and chains around the neck, and earrings, facial studs, etc.** These can be dangerous – confused or aggressive patients could grab and pull them.

- **Uniforms.** If the university says wear grey trousers, wear grey trousers. Wear your uniform according to the university policy. If you wear street clothes, make sure you are dressed appropriately. Football strips, tee-shirts with slogans, and stained or torn clothing all say 'I'm not very professional', and could upset vulnerable patients.

- **BE ON TIME.** If you know you can't get there on time because of child care or other obligations, then negotiate your schedule.

- **Visit the placement in advance.** When you find out the time and location of your placement, call and make an appointment to visit. Try to meet your mentor and/or some of the ward staff. Ask about shifts, parking, where to put your coat, if you need to bring your own cup/teabags, etc. Find out about the off-duty (when you are working). (You are not on the off-duty because you are counted in the numbers; it is for safety so people know where you should be and so your mentor can plan his or her workload.)

- **Know what happens in the placement area.** When you are scheduled for a particular placement area, prepare yourself. Don't be like a Miss America student who, when asked what she would like, said 'A general overview. And world peace'. Be specific. Think about the kinds of specialties and patients the ward will have, think about what interests you in the specialty and ask about it. Try to prepare for special terms! For example, if it's an ear, nose and throat (ENT) ward, get an ENT textbook out of the library, brush up on the anatomy and physiology of the ear, nose and throat, and try to learn some of the terms you will encounter. The nurses and staff there will have invested a lot in their specialty, and seeing a student motivated to learn about their kind of nursing will inspire them. That means a better placement for you.

- **Develop student 'antennae'.** Try to work out the best (and worst) times to approach your mentor or other staff nurses. It makes life easier for everyone – especially you. Just imagine . . . you are driving to work in the lovely brand new car you and your partner have saved so hard to buy. As the result of some rather unfortunate experiences, by the time you get home the car looks more like a piece of modern art than it did: it's a write-off. Your partner comes home late, looking rather flustered and upset – a bad day at the office. Is this the best moment to say: 'Darling, I crashed the car'? No, it's the best time to help your partner get through the crisis and then, when it's over, you can explain how you have a submission for the Turner Prize called 'Was once a car...' and how your partner now has a perfect opportunity to buy that other model he or she wanted. It's the same with your mentor.

- **Be sensitive to patient perspectives.** Patients will sometimes do or say things that really aren't acceptable in our culture – ridiculously biased things like 'I don't want a black nurse', 'You're too fat to be my nurse', or 'I don't want a male nurse, they're all gay'. Please, don't allow yourself to be abused, but try to remember that when people are ill they aren't themselves. Some patients will have wandering hands. Try not to over-react or be afraid. Be firm, but caring. Remember that your appearance may sometimes seem threatening to patients. If you have brightly dyed hair, a lot of facial piercings, and/or visible tattoos, there is a chance that some patients could react. I have even had people react to my American accent! They said things that were hurtful, although they didn't intend them to be that way. People who are ill are afraid, and people who are afraid often cope in very strange ways. If someone slips up and says something unkind or judgemental,, they are not reacting to you as a person: it's up to you to try to be therapeutic anyway. If someone abuses you, get support from your mentor and other nurses.

- **Be sensitive to staff.** Be aware of and respect policies, procedures and the chain of command in the area in which you are working. Try to think of yourself as an ambassador – your behaviour and attitude will affect the way future nursing students are treated. One student can ruin it for all the other students who follow, and can make things very difficult for staff. Do the best you can to respect the way staff do things.

We'll talk more about things as the chapter goes on, but if you remember nothing else, remember this:

Always be on time, neat, clean and dressed appropriately to make the best, most professional impression.

What kind of student are you?

You're probably tired of talking about nursing and placements, so let's take a minute to talk about something else . . .

Let's imagine that you are going on a wonderful holiday. You have been given a week-long adventure in Florida. You have been to a travel agent, who has given you a list of all the places you can visit. You have been told you will have a dedicated tour guide while you are there. You are leaving in 3 weeks. What do you do?

A. You wait for the tour guide to send you info, and aren't particularly bothered when he doesn't.
B. You ask friends who have been to Florida about their experiences.
C. You get brochures and maybe even a book to give you more information about the sights and ideas about what to do.

Your cases are packed and you are on your way. You get to your hotel, unpack and wait for your tour guide to show up. The office staff say that they are overbooked, so the tour guide is not coming today. In fact, they can't tell you when or if the tour guide is ever going to come. Do you:

A. Sit by the pool, not worrying that you only have a week and have a lot of things you would like to do.
B. Try to get something done that is on your list.
C. Call the travel agent and let them know that there is a problem.

The travel agent calls you and asks how things are going. You explain the tour guide situation and the agent tells you to go it alone today while he or she tries to do something for you. Do you:

A. Do nothing but get a sunburn waiting for someone to call you back.
B. Do something around the hotel – maybe *EastEnders* is on TV!
C. Do something nearby that is on your list.

Your tour guide, as a result of a short call from your travel agency, shows up the next day. He asks you what you would like to do. Do you:

A. Shrug your shoulders and say 'I dunno'.
B. Say 'Whatever you want me to will be OK with me'.
C. Grab your pamphlets and books and point out what interests you.

Your tour guide takes you to two places that day – one is rubbish and the other is the most wonderful and amazing place you have ever seen. The next day, when you have some free time, do you:

A. Complain to everyone about what kind of experience you had at the rubbish place.
B. Talk about how great the good place was.
C. Write about the good place – you want to remember all the details!

At the end of the holiday, you have had a great time. There are some people who really made a difference to you. The tour guide, once he showed up, was pretty amazing and really gave a lot extra. The clerk at the hotel was very friendly. Even the housekeeper treated you like her own child. What do you do?

A.   Leave a mess – after all they are paid to clean up after you – and mumble something that sounds like 'Thanks' as the taxi comes to take you to the airport.
B.   Think about how great everyone has been.
C.   Thank each person, and send a card to the hotel manager and tour guide agency telling them how good the experience was.

Your plane lands and you are walking through the airport. Everyone seems to be looking at you and there are television cameras; people are taking your picture. It seems your trip was part of a new reality television show ...

Looking back, were you the 'A' tourist – the one who waited for every experience to be inflicted on them, who complained and who had no initiative? Or were you the 'B' tourist – the one who made some effort, but didn't do much work? Or were you the 'C' tourist – the one who planned ahead, had initiative, showed real gratitude and took control of the holiday? The prize for the best contestant was a passing grade ... which of the three tourists do you think would win that coveted pass?

OK, that was a bit of fun, but in reality the difference between a rubbish clinical placement and a good one isn't really the mentor, the placement or even the other staff. It's all in how *you*, the student, approach what's before you. It's *your* placement.

What if things go wrong?

You have a number of options when there are problems on your placement:

- ignore them and hope they go away
- avoid them by calling in sick
- keep your head down and try just to live through it
- complain to everyone who will listen
- go to your university or the ward manager (or the clinical placement facilitator) and explain the problem, asking for help and support.

The sooner you flag a problem or ask for help, the more likely there is to be a good outcome for you. If you wait until you get your final assessment to complain about your mentor, it will look like you are trying to get out of a bad review and it's unlikely you will be taken seriously.

In the unlikely event that things start to go wrong, you need to do a few things:

- **Document!** Write down when things are said or done that aren't right. Keep a time line – when things happened, who did them, etc. Don't be in the situation where you have to say 'I don't know who told me, but . . .'
- **Reflect: what is really going wrong?** Is any of it your fault? Did you make things worse? What do you need to do differently? What do you need to go forward?
- **Make sure of the rules.** Check policies and university guidelines. Is it your perspective that is wrong, or is something being done improperly?

If you do need to complain, you have to know how:

- **Take an advocate**: your union, student union or university rep should be with you. Talk to them – they are used to complaining and sorting things out.
- **Use your time line** to show a clear history of the problem.
- **Be objective:** don't get personal. 'She hates me' is not a good place to start a complaint. Relate specific examples openly and honestly.
- **Be willing to work things out:** don't get stubborn or difficult. Express what is wrong and what you need, and try to be flexible.
- **Let go of the past:** if things are discussed and everyone makes plans to move forward, don't hold a grudge. Be a professional and be willing to give others a chance.

To summarize all this, remember: this is *your* placement. Your mentor, the ward manager and the other staff nurses have already passed their course. It's not up to you to worry about them; it's up to you to worry about you. If they don't do things the right way, then learn from their example anyway. You can learn from bad practice just as you can learn from good practice.

You may find yourself in a situation where you witness something you cannot ignore: a medication error, harm to a patient, theft or abuse. If that is the case, seek support from someone before bringing it forward. As a student you are vulnerable, and you must accept that there are times when you need support. Whistle-blowing is a serious issue and can be very stressful. You are obliged to blow the whistle if you witness something serious, and there are people at your university and in your union who are obliged to help you. Don't feel you have to go it alone. I can't really prepare you here for the stress and anxiety that whistle-blowing could potentially bring – if you know that some-thing must be brought out into the open, get support through your university, union or student union.

SUPERNUMERARY STATUS

> I know students are supposed to be supernumerary, but how are they going to learn to be nurses if they sit at the desk reading a magazine?
>
> *Mentor*

Supernumerary status is one of those things that has no real definition. What it means in theory is that you are not staff on the ward, so you do not have the same responsibilities and obligations. Whereas other staff members are there to take care of patients and meet the needs of the ward, you are there to meet your learning needs and objectives. This can conflict with the nature of clinical placements. On placement, you learn by 'being a nurse', by giving hands-on care and by pitching in as part of the team. There is a subtle, but important, difference – you:

- are there to learn
- must be supervised
- are there to help out as a team member to learn about the team and how it works
- must meet your learning outcomes
- must stay within the scope of your knowledge and skills as a student nurse.

You are not:

- there to staff the ward
- there to fulfil the role of any other nurse or nursing assistant in their absence
- there to supervise any patient in a one-to-one capacity (because you yourself need supervision)
- to put 'getting the work done' before your learning
- ever to step beyond the limitations of your role, no matter what you know from your past career and education
- to 'cover' the placement area without a nurse present.

It is difficult – the ward is down a nurse, and a healthcare assistant, and the patients are still in bed at 10 am. You want to go to see a diagnostic test being done on a patient you have been following all week. The sister tells you that you are needed to bathe patients and so you can't go. What do you do? There is no easy answer.

An isolated episode like this doesn't mean your supernumerary status has been compromised. I hope you never stand on a ward with your hands on your hips while patients are in need and say, 'I'm a student and I am not going to help'. You have to use your judgement. If it is happening all the time or you hear 'We don't need a healthcare assistant, we have a student...', then do something about it:

- document what is happening
- talk to the ward manager, your mentor, the university and your union as soon as you are aware of the problem
- don't just ignore it – other students and, most important, patients are affected.

So, points to remember about being supernumerary... Being supernumerary means:

- you are not there to replace, or to fill in for, a member of staff at any level
- you need to put your learning outcomes before the staffing needs of the placement area
- you do have a role as a member of the team on the placement area
- you have a responsibility to patients and families
- you must never act outside the scope of your education and student role
- you have the right to mentorship and support in meeting your learning outcomes
- you are *not* a nurse and you are *not* a healthcare assistant – you are a student who is there to learn while doing, and to practise essential skills to gain competency.

Ask yourself: Is this helping me become a good, competent nurse? Am I learning new skills and building on established ones? Am I getting chances to have new experiences and to grow as a nurse? If the answer is 'Yes', then you are probably OK.

There have always been concerns about students learning at the hands of non-teachers... Some of the placement areas don't assess the student well. Some of them don't teach the student. Some of them provide inadequate mentorship and so use the student as cheap labour. But what do all placements have in common? YOU!

The code of conduct clearly states that you have an obligation to recognize your limitations. OK, so as a student it doesn't strictly apply to you... but it's a big clue about what you should be doing in practice: don't just get by, excel. Don't just cover the basics; drench yourself in nursing and be as good as you can. You should figure out what you need to be fit as a nurse, then do everything you can to make sure you become that nurse. If you are not competent, don't sigh with relief when you don't get caught out – go and tell someone. How would you like it if an incompetent nurse were caring for someone you love?

BECOMING A NURSE ONE PLACEMENT AT A TIME

You are becoming a nurse, one placement at a time. You have an obligation to become that nurse – but it will also make your course more enjoyable if you plot your own progress. Your university will give you ample pieces of paper to fill out to chart your progress, but I will bet that you yourself won't see that inner nurse emerging.

First, I would like to challenge you to learn about **ACT A PUP**. This is a mnemonic to help you remember what you are trying to accomplish – key elements of nursing. At the end of this chapter there is a placement checklist; it has a number of reflections, but this is the one you can easily use as often as needed. To show yourself how much you are growing, try to reflect on the following, every day, every week and for every placement.

In this placement, how have I demonstrated that I:
- – am trustworthy
- – communicate in a professional manner
- – technically am a competent nurse
- – act as a role model and good example for students and junior staff
- – put my patients first
- – use appropriate infection control skills
- – practise safely, with appropriate manual handling skills.

By doing this, you will be constantly looking not just to the end of the module, the placement, the year, but to how you need to carry yourself as a nurse.

It is also helpful for you to identify what models of nursing people are using, and to start to develop comfort with one particular nursing model. If you know one model well, you can use it to guide you in your practice. Try to assess patients on your own before you read how others have assessed them, and see what you missed and what you found. Don't be afraid to ask questions: get out there and start thinking!

MENTORSHIP

When you start a placement, you will be assigned a mentor. This person assesses you and will sign off your competencies. She will usually have undertaken a mentorship and assessors course.

If you plan a pre-placement visit to the placement area, you really should try to meet your mentor. You will probably follow a similar off-duty (work schedule) to your mentor, to make sure you have ample time to work together. You should work with your mentor at least two shifts a week. Busy placement areas will often assign you a mentor and a 'back-up' mentor, so that you have the best support, and to take the pressure off staff. Your mentor is there to:

- make sure you meet the required competencies to pass the placement
- be your teacher and supervisor
- make certain you comply with policies like manual handling
- fulfil the requirement that someone qualified to be a mentor is present in placement areas where there are students.

Your mentor is also there to do a number of other things:

- staff the ward
- do paperwork
- take care of patients
- take care of families
- resolve complaints and staff issues
- do the off duty
- answer the phone
- pass medications
- do treatments and dressings
- monitor patients
- respond to consultants' and doctors' requests and orders
- do care planning . . .

. . . I'm sure you get the hint: your mentor is a busy nurse. Often, your mentor will be a ward sister (or charge nurse), the busiest of all the ward nurses on any given shift. How can you and this nurse make the best of this important relationship?

- **Have a clue.** Go into your placement knowing what you need to accomplish, and have some idea of how you plan to accomplish your goals and outcomes. Read about the placement area before you go in. What kind of nursing is it? What kinds of patients will there be?
- **Be a good team member.** Respect the fact that sister (or the charge nurse) may have pressing things to accomplish. Don't wait for her to approve your every move – the rest of the team from domestic to HCA to staff nurse all has knowledge you can make use of. Build a good network for yourself.
- **Know the deadlines.** Be assertive about getting your paperwork done. 'Sister, I need my assessment done by Friday. Can we schedule some time please? I've already done my part . . .'. Don't wait for her to psychically determine that you are ready for your assessment. It's *your* assessment,

you need to make sure it gets done. Don't wait until the end of your placement – make sure your assessments are done when they are due.

- **Communicate.** Tell your mentor or other staff nurse when you are having problems. Ask for help when you need it. Let someone know if something is going wrong, as soon as possible. You have a lot of resources – union reps, student union, placement facilitators, university staff, personal tutors, ward managers; if something is going wrong and you don't tell anyone, it is no one's fault but yours when your mentor fails you.

- **Get along.** Not everyone is compatible with everyone else. You will have mentors who don't like you and you will have mentors you don't like. You might not agree with them; you might just be so different as individuals that you can't see eye to eye. Be professional and do the best you can to get along. This doesn't mean you should allow yourself to be bullied or mistreated; it just means that you shouldn't expect every mentor to be your best friend. Learning to get along with different kinds of people is essential to nursing; it's yet another lesson you can learn from your student–mentor relationship.

- **Be professional.** Don't *ever* do things you are not qualified to do. Don't cover up mistakes. Ask for help when you need it. Be cheerful and pleasant, and don't gossip

- **Consider your achievements and make sure you have proven that you are achieving as required to go to the next level.** Is there anything from this placement that could serve as evidence; anything here that would benefit your progress to achievement; any new skills that you could learn; any established skills that you could build on; any skills that you could develop in a slightly different way than before, showing you have more than one dimension to your skill?

- **Use 'student antennae'.**

Your mentor should make sure that your placement gives you skills and experience. Sometimes that won't work quite the way you want it to. By working cooperatively with the placement area staff and being responsible for yourself, you give your assessment the best foundation it can have. Ultimately, it is up to you – your conduct, your behaviour, your skills – to make sure you pass your placement.

OTHER PEOPLE WHO HELP YOU LEARN

There are some other people who will support you during your placement:

- **Clinical placement coordinator.** This is a nurse who oversees where students are placed and what kinds of rotations they have. Her job is to make sure that you have a placement, that there are mentors, and that no one area is overwhelmed. She organizes intakes from different universities. Her job is to make sure that every student has a mentor and a good placement, and that any problems are identified and resolved.

- **Link tutor.** This is a tutor who comes from your university and connects with you and other nurses in the area. Her job is to help solve any problems that arise, as well as to make sure that you are being correctly assessed by the mentor.
- **Clinical tutor/clinical educator.** This is a nurse who has special training that allows her to teach people clinical skills in the clinical environment. She might work for your university, or she might work for the clinical area. It's not up to her necessarily to assess you, but she might help your mentor assess you properly.

Summary

It all boils down to AAA:

- **Attendance:** show up on time and only take a sick day if you truly need it
- **Appearance:** look the part of a professional nurse
- **Attitude:** have a smile on your face, be positive and don't complain when things go wrong – look for solutions.

If you want to be taken seriously as a professional nurse, look like one. Be:

- neat
- clean (and without excess make-up and jewellery)
- on time.

There are different branches in nursing, and you will have placements in the different branch areas. If you decide you want to go into a different branch, you can negotiate to change branches – but there needs to be a good reason, and there needs to be 'room' in the branch into which you want to transfer. Don't plan on such a transfer being easy.

Remember that:

- Your placements are there to develop you into a competent qualified nurse.
- You need to be an active and eager participant in your education and development.

- You may need to complain, seek help or blow the whistle. Make sure you know the contact details of the people who are there to help you at your union, your student union, your university, and the trust in which you are placed.

- You need to be progressing towards achievement of the ESCs, either towards branch or towards registration.

- You are supernumerary, but that doesn't mean that you sit around waiting to be taught something; it also means that you do not replace paid staff. Being a team member is essential to learning how to be a competent nurse. You are there to get your learning outcomes met and to become more competent.

- Your mentor will be a busy nurse with many responsibilities. Be considerate and know what you need for help and support.

- Be prepared to be assertive – but also understanding – about getting your needs met.

- It's *your* placement, *your* portfolio, *your* pass. Know your portfolio and assessment documents and take responsibility for getting things done.

One note – I had a lovely student named Gillian. She at first disliked the placement area – it was not very exciting, involving a lot of hard, fundamental care and not a lot of technology or excitement. Then, she recognized the value of the fundamental care. She went on to write a fabulous paper on the placement area – one which affected not only the staff and the hospital, but also her own tutor. She recognized that patients need nurses who have excellence in the most fundamental things, and that her achievement on the placement was to understand the value of 'basic care'.

Gillian's gift to the ward was not just her praise; her paper will also be used to teach others. She lifted morale, helped the ward establish a more dominant role in the service, and made herself look like a star in the process. Don't underestimate the amount of power you have – the assessment you make of the clinical area will carry weight and can make a difference. If you have had a good placement, say so. If it has been bad, explain why and give precise explanations. If people helped you, name them. If they made life hell, name them too. If you don't say what happened, no one can make it better . . . and if you don't praise those staff who helped you, they may not see the value in helping others. You like praise and positive feedback too, right?

In closing, I ask you please to remember the reason you are on placement: it is to build skills and knowledge, by caring for actual patients. Patients don't know you are a student – they trust you. You owe it to them to do your best, but also to own up to it when you can't do something. You owe it to patients to help them trust other staff; although it feels good when a patient *only* wants to talk to you, you need to help them have others to talk to, too. Don't do anything that will make them lose trust in the staff or the care they are receiving.

Look at the sections in Chapter 6 on assertiveness and the other skills essential to surviving placements and nurse education – not skills like taking a blood pressure or passing a nasogastric tube, but skills like how to stand up for yourself!

> I'm a mentor now and every time my student nurse frustrates me, I try to think back to when I was a student. I remember being a student nurse and thinking, 'When did my mentor develop such amnesia about being a student nurse herself?' It helps me be a little more patient and understanding about how difficult it can be to be a student nurse. I just wish the student could understand how hard it can be to be a mentor!
>
> *Nurse, qualified 3 years*

REFERENCES

Department of Health, 1999. Making a Difference. HMSO, London
UKCC, 1999. Fitness for Practice (the Peach Report). UKCC, London

Placement checklist (you can download a copy from the Evolve website http://evolve.elsevier.com/siviter/studentnurse/)

Placement area: _____ Location: _____

Correct uniform: any changes from usual?

Time day shift starts: _____ Time shift ends: _____

Time of evening shift: _____ Shift ends: _____

Time night shift ends: _____ Shift ends: _____

What type of patients are found in this clinical area?

Mentor name: _____ Contact: _____

Date of first interview: _____

Date of second interview: _____

Date of final interview: _____ Placement ends: _____

First day on the ward/clinical area: I need to know: _____

- [ ] Fire exits and fire routine: what is the emergency number to dial?
- [ ] What are the possible roles I might have if there were a fire?
- [ ] How to get emergency help for a patient: what is the right number?
- [ ] Names of area manager and mentor: Manager: _____
- [ ] What to do if I need to call in sick: Clinical area telephone: _____
- [ ] Location of the toilet, staff room and where I can store my things
- [ ] When breaks take place
- [ ] Where I can get lunch/dinner/drinks

- [ ] The best parking area or the best place to get a bus
- [ ] Clinical area's philosophy
- [ ] Location of clinical policy folder
- [ ] Location of health and safety information
- [ ] Are there any infection control or health and safety risks present?
- [ ] Location of student resource information
- [ ] Where is off duty kept/how to request time
- [ ] Telephone number for Clinical Placement Coordinator

Any other information: door codes, etc.

During placement:

What skills do I need to develop during this placement?

How can I support staff in this area while maintaining boundaries?

Identify at least one good role model: what is it about that nurse that makes him or her a good nurse? How can I be more like them?

What did I do well and what should I have done differently?

On reflection, in this placement, have I demonstrated that I:
- am trustworthy
- communicate in a professional manner
- technically am a competent nurse
- act as a role model and good example for students and junior staff
- put my patients first
- use appropriate infection control skills
- practise safely, with appropriate manual handling skills

At end of placement checklist:

☐ Thank you note or card to placement area and to mentor

☐ Honest feedback about placement area to university

☐ Approach people who have made a real difference to me and thank them

☐ Decide what I am going to keep from this placement and plan on how to integrate into practice

☐ Apologize to any staff if necessary

☐ Return anything I borrowed

On reflection, in what areas have I grown during this placement, and in what areas do I still need to develop?

Basics of Nursing

5

In this chapter

- Basic nursing qualities
- Vignettes
- Communication skills

As a nurse, there are some basic skills you will need. As a student, you must actively develop these skills from the first day you enter your course. Some will be obvious – manual handling, for example – but some won't. You will be changing the way you think and act as you learn more about nursing and health care.

It is a good idea to, from the very start, think and act with an awareness of how you want to be as a nurse. This is much easier said than done, but, like any practical skill or habit, practise makes perfect.

These basic skills are the same, although adapted, no matter which branch of nursing you are in. You can earn your pay regardless, but in my opinion (and in the opinion of the patient's association) you won't be a nurse without them. So, what are they?

I'll start with a brief list, then talk about a few situations that explain their value before giving you a few more tools and concepts that will help it all make sense. Although none of the vignettes and examples here is based on word-for-word patient experiences or individual people, they are all based on things I have experienced as a nurse or patient myself. They are truthful and real, but blended so that no one's confidentiality is broken. Names are made up.

BASIC NURSING QUALITIES

- **Empathy.** This is caring about what happens to people. It is different from sympathy, where you care about people and feel badly for them; empathy is when you can put yourself in someone else's place, and approach that person's care as if you were thinking about the kind of care you would want for yourself or those you love.

- **Communication skills.** Communication comes in different forms. You can talk, but what do you say? You can hear, but do you listen? You can write, but does it matter? It's not just what you say, write or read; it's how . . . your body language and style will say much more than your actual words.

- **Nursing theory.** You need a foundation in nursing theory so you can approach care, assessment, care planning and delivery, and evaluation of care from a nursing perspective. Nursing is a unique and special profession, not because of the tools we use, but because of the way we use them. How we think, what we look for, and how we approach care . . . this is the foundation of nursing.

- **Compassion.** Compassion is when you feel for others, where the suffering or discomfort of another person affects you. It's related to empathy but slightly different – it's not just caring, but feeling like you can't ignore someone else's problems.

- **Common sense.** This means being able to think about things and have some 'street sense' – a way of relating to people, to situations and to experiences that reflects insight.

- **Organization.** You have to be able to prioritize and organize your work as a nurse, and it starts with your student days. There will always be a lot to get done, and you have to get the most important things done first. Someone's life could depend on your ability to do the right things at the right time.

- **Critical thinking.** This is the ability to question things, to stop and say 'What, how am I sure it's this and not that?'; being careful not to make assumptions, or take things for granted.

- **Fearlessness.** OK, maybe that's not quite the right way to say it, but you need to not worry about how your colleagues will react, or if they won't like you because you do something a certain way; the only person whose opinion matters to you should be your patient. Even if you get stick from someone else, you should never be afraid to do the right thing for your patient.

- **Reflection.** You must be willing to look at yourself and your practice, and constantly think 'Is this right? Is it enough? Should I change?' Nursing is not a profession where you can settle in to a certain way and be confident that it will always be the right way. Things change, and you need to be ready to change too.

Let's look at the difference some of these skills can mean for patients.

VIGNETTES

Let's do lunch

Angela, one of your senior colleagues, is telling you how her shift on the overnight went:

> That guy John, admitted with persistent nausea? First of all, the pharmacy never sent up his meds, and then, he was sick all over my uniform. Can

you believe it? People like that – I mean, couldn't he use a bowl? He was so impatient . . . he woke up everyone in the bay . . . he was one of those 'nurse, nurse wipe my brow' types, you know, the ones who like the attention of being sick? I had to have someone else bring my lunch back, after spending so much time waiting on him and then cleaning my uniform . . .

This is the way John saw it:

I had a terrible night. I was sick all night, they never brought in the injection the doctor said I would have. I called for the nurse because I dropped the last bowl I had to use and was just too weak to get up. I called and called, but no one came, and I was so afraid and worried . . . I wouldn't usually ask for help, but what could I do? Three of us were awake anyway, the staff had been laughing and talking out in the corridor. When I called and no one came, the man in the bed next to me pushed his call light, too.

When the nurse finally came, she had such an attitude – here I am, sick, and she couldn't just take a few minutes and worry about me rather than herself? Why did she have to start carrying on about bacon sandwiches and such while I am there green and sick? She was the coldest, least compassionate person I ever met. What is she at work for if not to help? I'm sorry I interrupted her conversation, but, that's why I was in hospital!'

'Do you really want to hurt me?'

Todd, the nurse, is giving you handover from the morning:

Arlene, Bed 2, this woman – well, she is a real attention seeker. She is obese, does as little as possible, and really likes her pain medication. Try to make her wait before just medicating her – she doesn't look like she is in pain, and we shouldn't just give in to those kinds of behaviours. Also, try to make her do more for herself – don't offer help until she has really pushed herself.

Arlene calls her daughter while the nurses are in handover:

Cathy, get me out of here. The nurses – they think I am lying. I can hardly move, but they wouldn't help me get washed or dressed, and they made me wait over an hour for my pain medication and I wet myself waiting for help to get up to the toilet. They admitted me because my mobility is so poor, hoping physio could help get these old joints moving again, but no one will help me!

I can't cope – I am am trying to keep a stiff upper lip, even though it hurts so bad, but if they are going to be like this I need to get out of here. One of the nurses even said 'come on now, are you really in pain?' Doesn't she know that once you have been in pain for 12 years, I've gotten really good at not letting the pain show? Shouldn't the nurse be experienced enough to know? That, and when they finally did help me, the two nurses washing me chit-chatted back and forth like they were washing a car or something. They just ignored me, like I was an inconvenience . . . . Either come get me or I am going to call a taxi . . .

What went wrong?

What has happened in both of these vignettes? It sounds like the nurse and the patient were in completely different places! In these cases, the nurse approached the patient not as a *nurse* should but as another *person* would. When you are a nurse, you can't be the same as you are when you are off duty. You have to put your own needs, perceptions, beliefs and biases aside. You have to be there for patients, as their advocate, and with them at the centre of everything you do. You should see patients as the experts, and not expect them to prove that they are truthful. You must be patient, kind, and helpful, even if you think a person is taking advantage of you. It's not up to you to judge; it's up to you to care.

In 'Let's do lunch', the nurse was busy, and angry at the patient for needing her when it was time for her lunch. Why didn't she make sure the patient had his medication? Why were people so loud in the corridor? And since when do you talk about food in front of someone who is sick? She blamed the patient, and didn't take any accountability for her own actions. She couldn't see how her actions affected the patient. Maybe she was too tired, or maybe it was a bad night, but that's not the patient's fault.

In 'Do you really want to hurt me', the nurse was too inexperienced to know the difference between acute and chronic pain. Chronic pain – in reality, chronic illness in general – doesn't show the way acute pain or illness does; people get used to it, and develop coping skills that hide it. They can't get on with life if they are miserable every day, so they learn to accept their discomfort and do the best they can.

The nurse needs not only to assess the pain, and patients' ability to care for themselves, based on what they say, but also to take the patients' word for what their needs and abilities are. All Arlene needed was for the nurse to accept her complaints at face value, and treat her accordingly.

Another thing that went wrong in 'Did you really want to hurt me' was that the nurses didn't involve the patient in her care. When you are washing or caring for someone with a colleague, it's easy to carry on chatting to the colleague – but that makes the patient feel like an object. How does that help patients trust you, believe in you, and feel like you understand them? It doesn't– but the Code of Conduct says you must do all those things. Improving your nursing communication skills is the best way to make sure that you can provide the care and support your patients need.

COMMUNICATION SKILLS

There are three actual different types of communication:

1. Verbal communication
2. Non-verbal communication (body language)
3. Written communication.

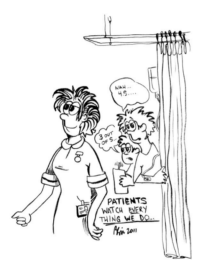

In this section, we are going to talk about how to communicate in a positive, non-threatening way. As nurses, we have specific ways of communicating, we have words 'regular' people don't use, we have short cuts when we write – but in spite of all that, let me tell you a secret . . . sometimes, nurses don't really communicate well.

- We interrupt patients when they talk to us:
  Patient: 'I miss my husband so much . . .'
  Nurse: 'Yes, Mrs Brown, did someone take your blood pressure?'
- We explain things instead of just listening:
  Patient: 'I have so much pain'
  Nurse: 'Well, after surgery, everyone does'.

○ We make judgements:

Nurse writes on assessment document, under 'sexuality', 'deferred' because the patient is over 50

Nurse sees a young, single mother with several young children and assumes she is on benefits.

○ We avoid discussion we can't handle:

Patient: 'I am worried I am dying'

Nurse: 'Now, now, don't worry about that. Let's see, which jumper would you like to wear?'

○ We treat patients like they are 'work' rather than people:

(Nurses washing patient who has been inpatient for 3 weeks) 'So, what are you doing after work?' 'I want to go to the mall, but Jack might call me so I don't know yet. Have you seen that new movie with Brad Pitt? I can't wait to get out of this place today. Roll over so I can wash your back, OK?'

○ We focus on tasks and can see talking to patients as an interruption or a waste of time:

Patient: 'Nurse, if I could just talk to you for a minute . . .'

Nurse: 'What do you need?'

Patient: 'Well, I just wanted to talk . . . '

Nurse: 'I am far too busy for conversation, but if I have a chance, I'll get back to you.'

Here's an example about communication – it was also in the last edition of this book. A student came up to me at an event and said 'You know that example about Mr Brown and communication? When I first read it, before my course, I thought 'That would never happen', but on my very first day of placement, I heard something nearly identical . . . . I don't ever want to be that kind of nurse.' I hope you strive to be a better nurse than this, too.

Verbal communication

Mr Brown

Mr Brown is in bed, and the nurse is bringing linen to all the bedsides in preparation for bed changes.

Mr Brown: 'Nurse, I'm really worried that I'm not getting any better.'

Nurse: 'Oh, Mr Brown, you look great today . . .' (keeps putting linen by beds)

Mr Brown: 'Yes, OK . . .' (looks away)

What is Mr Brown really trying to say? He's saying 'Nurse, I'm afraid . . . .' How does the nurse reply? Basically, by saying 'Buzz off, I'm busy'. Now, it's okay to be busy – nurses are busy people and getting busier all the time – but how would it be if it went this way instead for Mr Brown?

> Mr Brown: 'Nurse, I'm really worried that I'm not getting any better.'
>
> Nurse: (stops what she is doing) 'Mr Brown, you have been unwell a long time and it must feel as though it's never going to get any better' (gives Mr Brown's hand a quick squeeze)
>
> Mr Brown: 'Yes, I have been ill so long – am I dying and no one told me?'
>
> Nurse: 'Mr Brown, I don't think you are dying, but I can imagine it's very frustrating to be unwell for so long. Would you like me to ask the doctor to talk to you about how long it is taking to get better?'
>
> Mr Brown: 'If it's not too much trouble . . .'
>
> Nurse: 'Not at all, Mr Brown, as soon as I am done with the linen, I will put it in the doctor's book. And Mr Brown? Thanks for asking me . . . if you want to talk some more, let me know.'

See the difference? In the second example, the nurse does something called 'reflecting'. She takes Mr Brown's words and rephrases them, repeating them back to show what she heard and to give him permission to continue. The nurse shows she takes him seriously, and gives him a reasonable expectation of what she will do. She then also invites him to come back to her if he needs more help. How differently would Mr Brown feel in the second example than in the first? How would you want someone you love spoken to?

Improving communication

There are some basic ways we can improve our communication as nurses. None of these takes a long time; in fact, some of them will save you time in the long run because you will resolve a problem rather than letting it get worse. Best of all, these are all ways of keeping your patient central to everything you do.

- **Be honest.** If you can't help Mr Brown right now, tell him– but, also tell him when you will be able to help him
- **Keep your promises.** If you say you will come back, or do something, then do as you said or come back and explain why you didn't. Get someone else to help you if needed, but don't leave the patient waiting.
- **You don't have to fix everything.** Sometimes, people just want to know that someone else is there, they aren't looking for a solution, they just don't want to feel alone.
- **There is nothing such as a right or wrong 'feeling'.** It's OK if you and a patient see a situation differently. If Mr Brown says 'You ignored me', the right answer is 'I'm sorry you feel that way', not 'No I didn't'. Don't argue with patients. You don't have to be right, and to be honest, it's the patient's opinion that matters most.

- **A little empathy goes a long way.** It doesn't cost you anything to have a bit of compassion and empathy for what people are going through. Feeling bad that someone is in pain, or that they had to wait for care – and telling the person – can help build trust between you.

- **It's not about you.** Sometimes people we care for, or those who care about them, can be unpleasant, aggressive and rude. Try to be understanding and patient: don't let yourself be abused, but try to see things from the other person's point of view. People are coping with pain, fear, or might be confused or affected by their illness or medication – nurses don't see them at the easiest moments of their lives. Take a deep breath and don't take things personally: 99 per cent of the time, they aren't really angry with you, they are angry with circumstances. How would you be feeling if you had to cope with all the things the people you care for have to cope with? Getting angry back only makes it worse, and makes it impossible for you to provide nursing care.

- **Smile, touch, laugh, cry, be yourself.** As long as you keep your boundaries, use good judgement, and always act in your patient's best interest – show your feelings. A friend once said 'You can always tell the best nurses – they are the ones who cry . . .' What he meant was that good nurses aren't cold or distant about the work they do. People who are ill want to be cared for by people, not machines. The real exception to this is when you are caring for people who have a mental illness or learning disability that could result in them misinterpreting your intentions. You don't want to give the wrong message; you do, however, want to show that you *care*.

- **Don't treat patients as if they aren't there.** Don't talk to your friend when you make Mr Brown's bed; talk to *him*. Don't chat to someone else when you are taking his observations, it will hurt his feelings. He's stuck in the hospital worried about getting better, and he hears you chatting about your big night out – how do you think it makes him feel? Take opportunities to communicate. And what about Mrs Cecile, who has had a stroke and is unconscious? Talk to her, too. Maybe, just maybe, she can hear you. You might be the only person who speaks to her all day. How long could you go through life without anyone talking to you – not at you or just around you?

- **Explain things.** How would you feel if you were in bed, couldn't see, couldn't talk, couldn't move, and all of a sudden someone was washing your genitals? Try to put yourself in the patient's place. Ask permission, even if the person is unconscious. 'Mr Akram, I'd like to give you a bath, OK?' A small thing can make such a difference. It's respectful.

○ **Be polite.** Say 'please', 'thank you' and 'excuse me'. Address people by their surname (Mr, Mrs, Miss) until told otherwise. Introduce yourself. Ask permission. Don't assume Mr Akram will allow you to call him Ronnie; ask him if you may.

○ **Don't force a patient to interrupt your conversation with your colleague.** As soon as patients are near or approaching, make eye contact to let them know they have your full attention. Don't make them wait – you can talk to your friend anytime.

○ **Talk is therapy, just like medicine.** You don't need to be a professional counsellor to talk to patients; just listen and be a friend (a friend with good boundaries!). Make sure, however, that you stay within the scope of your role.

○ **Keep your body language open.** Smile, make eye contact, don't tower over people when you speak to them, use touch when appropriate.

○ **Speak plainly.** 'Mrs Gardner, despite the complication of peritonitis after your laparoscopic appendectomy, the registrar feels that your course of cephalothin is resolving this and your prognosis is improving.' Do you think Mrs Gardner understood that? Why not just say 'The antibiotics we are giving you are helping and you are getting better'. Don't call the patient's jaw a 'mandible'; call it a 'jaw'. If you must use big words to impress your friends and family, fair enough, but always speak at the level you know the patient will understand. Make sure the patient and his or her family knows they can stop and ask you what something means. Don't ever tell a patient something that you don't understand the meaning of!

Good communication isn't difficult . . . so why don't we all do it? Maybe we are very task-oriented, and talking to the patient gets in the way of getting 'real' work done. Sometimes patients and families talk about things that we can't fix, and it's scary for us professional 'fixers' to be faced with not being able to do anything. Maybe we don't like people and we just don't want to be with them. In truth, sometimes we are genuinely busy and really don't have time.

Body language

Research says our body language communicates most of what others perceive. Now in some cases, that clearly isn't the truth – sometimes, it is the words that matter. 'FIRE!' doesn't rely on body language to communicate the problem – although, even then, that we are pointing in a direction gives important information. In regular conversation, however, it's not what we say, it's how – our expression, our posture, our eyes, the way we hold our hands . . . . To really control our communication, we must be aware of body language.

Basic body-language don'ts:

- Don't cross your arms across your chest– it looks like a barrier, and communicates aggressiveness.
- Don't cock your hip– you know that stance when one knee is a little bent and the other is straight? It says ' you are wasting my time'.
- Don't put your arms akimbo (that means on your hips with your elbows sticking out, but it was such a good word I had to use it) – it says 'yeah, yeah, when are you going to tell me something important'.
- Don't point at people when you speak to them.
- Don't look up or roll your eyes when others speak to you.
- Don't make gestures like rolling your hand to speed someone up when they are speaking.
- Don't stop someone from speaking with a 'stop' hand.

Important dos:

- Do remember to make eye contact when you talk to people.
- Do stop what you are doing and focus your body to mirror the other person's position when possible (clearly, if they are lying in bed you can't do that).
- Do move so that you are level with the other person. Therapeutic talking needs both people to be at the same physical level. You can't show how compassionate you are if you are towering over the other person.
- Do smile and nod when someone tells you something happy or good.
- Do sigh and shake your head when someone tells you something sad.
- Do use basic touch – hold a hand, pat on the shoulder – but don't use it in a demeaning or belittling way (more about that in a minute).
- Do explain if you need to hold a certain posture that you know can be perceived as aggressive. For example, when I sit, I cross my arms because it supports my back. I say 'Sorry for crossing my arms, but it hurts my back less – is it OK?'

If you want to let a person know you are really listening, there are some very specific active listening techniques. Active listening is what we do when another person is discussing things, one to one or in a meeting. It's a little different when you are interviewing or assessing someone – but I will explain the difference after this part.

There are six key aspects of active listening:

- **Be attentive.** Give a person your undivided attention. Look at his or her face without uncomfortable eye contact. Don't think about what you want to say or will say next – just listen. Look at a person's body language, and mirror it as much as possible. If you are in a group, don't indulge in side conversations or making comments when someone else is speaking.

- **Reflect.** Summarize what the other person is saying and repeat it back to him or her; this both shows that you are listening and gives the other person a chance to clarify anything that is misunderstood. Ask questions to clarify points or get the other person to expand on things. If in a group, raise your hand or respectfully interrupt if you need to ask for clarification: do this only if you can't allow the speaker to continue without the interruption. Try to think how you would feel in the other person's circumstances; this will help you let go of your own biases.

- **Turn off your filters.** Don't look for mistakes or places where you can correct the other person. Don't judge and accept things at face value. Just listen without an agenda or plan. Don't plan your argument while the other person is speaking; just listen.

- **Be an active listener.** Show that you are listening. Give verbal encouragements like 'Yes', 'really?' or 'uh huh' that say 'tell me more!' Use appropriate facial expressions and body language encouragements. Check your own body language, to remain open and available.

- **Zip your lip.** Aside from comments or questions meant to encourage the other person, don't say anything. Don't correct, don't argue, don't interrupt; just let the other person have his or her say. Wait for your turn to give your point of view. Don't rush others.

- **Use the 'Golden Rule'.** Treat the other person as you would want to be treated. Be respectful and honest, do not attack the other person, do not be derisive or make it hard for the other person.

It's not easy being an active listener. It takes a lot of concentration and determination to be an active listener. Old habits are hard to break, and if your listening habits are as bad as many people's are, then there's a lot of habit-breaking to do!

Be deliberate with your listening and remind yourself frequently that your goal is to truly hear what the other person is saying. Set aside all other thoughts and behaviours, and concentrate on the message. Ask questions, reflect, and paraphrase to ensure you understand the message. If you don't, then you'll find that what someone says to you and what you hear can be amazingly different!

Start using active listening today to become a better communicator, improve your workplace productivity, and develop better relationships.

6

Tools of the Trade

In this chapter

- Assertiveness
- Boundaries
- Coping with stress
- Delegation and organization
- Ethics
- Leadership
- Norms
- Governance
- Standards: essence of care and standards for better health
- References

ASSERTIVENESS

What is assertiveness?

- Respecting the rights and feelings of others while taking care of yourself
- Standing up for yourself and your rights
- Making clear what you want and need in a respectful way
- Being honest with yourself and others about what you need, what you can do, and how you are feeling
- Expressing your needs in a way that focuses on solutions.

Being assertive isn't the same as being a bully – when you behave in an assertive way, you shouldn't be hurting people's feelings or making people upset. Assertiveness doesn't include any of the following:

- blaming, shaming or name-calling
- unreasonable demands
- being manipulative
- anger, shouting or violence
- gossiping, backstabbing or prejudice.

Are you assertive?

I think most people would say they struggle to be assertive, but it's really an essential skill for a good nurse. It requires practice and reflection to develop assertiveness skills.

Some common feelings can get in the way when people try to be assertive. Remember that other people feel the same as you do when they try to be assertive – even people who seem really confident and self-assured. I'm a very assertive person, but sometimes I have to take a deep breath and overcome some very big butterflies in my guts when asserting myself! At some time or another, everyone feels afraid:

- that others will reject them
- that they will do something stupid
- of being embarrassed
- of losing friends or being gossiped about.

It's not just you who feels this way! But it can be very scary to assert yourself, especially when the person you are confronting is more powerful or more knowledgeable than you, or is aggressive. This is why you should be assertive even when it is scary:

- If you don't, you will feel upset that you didn't stand up for yourself
- If you let people take advantage of you, they will continue until you stand up to them or they grind you down
- If you can't take care of yourself, you can't hope to take care of anyone else (like patients!)
- Feeling used, disrespected, taken advantage of and powerless to speak up leads to stress and unhappiness
- By asserting yourself, you could change things for the better for everyone – chances are you are not the only person feeling the way you do!

Of course, there are some times when you can't assert yourself: 'Excuse me, I understand that you have had a lot to drink, but would you mind putting that machete down? It's making me very nervous.' If being assertive isn't going to get you anywhere, don't try it!

How do you frame an assertive confrontation?

1. **State the problem** (remember, stick to objective explanations, no feelings, no blame, no shame)
2. **State what you need and expect**

3. **Show the shared value in getting a good resolution**
4. **Know your limits,** and think about what you will do if the person with whom you are asserting yourself won't work with you.

For example: You get the off-duty and find that you are scheduled to work the weekend. Again. This is the third weekend in a row. You go to see the person who does the off-duty (note that although students are supernumerary, they are still scheduled on the off-duty so that their support can be planned; this is not meant to infer that students should not be supernumerary).

What you need to do

State the problem: 'I have seen the off-duty, and I am scheduled to work this weekend. I have worked the past two weekends in a row.'

State what you need: 'I should have this weekend off. I believe I have done my share.'

Show the shared value: 'I don't mind doing my share when I see the shifts are covered fairly.'

Know your limits: Have a plan for what to do if the person doesn't see that having you work all the weekends is a problem – see the ward manager, talk to the union steward, etc.

The person you are confronting could respond in a number of ways:

The response	Your reaction
'I'm sorry, I made a mistake, I'll fix it'	'I thought it was something like that, thanks for taking care of it' (Smile!)
'I'm sorry, I made a mistake, but it's too late to schedule someone else'	Is it worth arguing here? Either stick to your guns ('I am not working') or offer a reasonable alternative ('I'll work, but I'd like the next 4 weekends in a row off to make up for the weekends I have worked')
'I'm the one who does the off-duty, if you don't like it, tough!'	'Thank you for explaining this to me; I will need to discuss this with the ward manager' – then *go* to the ward manager
'No one else can work so I have to schedule you'	'I am not able to work every weekend; I feel weekends are something we all should share' – then go to see the ward manager and ask for help

It's easier to handle the response you might get if you think about it in advance. In this case, you would need to know in advance what kinds of alternatives you were willing to accept. Planning for a 'win–win' scenario (where each side gets some benefit) is important in making a good assertive confrontation. Think: what are the end results that you would be willing to accept?

A few points:

- **Be positive:** smile, be calm and don't overreact.
- **Always act as if a problem is the result of a misunderstanding or honest mistake:** this way, even if it was intentional, the other person has a graceful way out. If you back people into a corner, they will fight: it's not worth it.
- **Don't be passive-aggressive:** passive-aggressive behaviour is what happens when people are afraid of being angry, so they show their anger in a way that doesn't *look* angry. In the example above, if you had to work the weekend anyway, a passive-aggressive behaviour would be to call in sick. Gossiping about the person who did the off-duty, getting even by scheduling them for 3 weeks of weekends when you do the off-duty, getting revenge in sneaky ways – these are all passive-aggressive behaviours. Don't act that way.
- **Don't be manipulated:** people will react to confrontations in different ways, and they may act one way while really meaning something else. 'Oh, sorry, I thought it was your weekend to work, I'll take care of it for next week, promise' could mean 'You caught me, but I'm not doing anything about it, and if I can get away with it this time I'll probably try it again . . .'. Although you should try to accept what a person is doing and saying at face value, pay attention and be aware that there could be other factors at work. It would be OK to say 'I'm sure it was a mistake, but it is not my weekend, and I don't feel I should have to work it.'
- **Focus on solutions, not on blame/shame:** have some solutions and alternatives in mind when you start the confrontation.
- **Say how you are feeling:** start statements with 'I feel . . .', 'I want . . .' and 'I need . . .', not 'You do . . .' or 'You make me . . .'. Don't put words in people's mouths. Don't say 'We all . . .' or 'Everyone thinks . . .'. If you are the one asserting yourself, then speak only for yourself unless you are there as a member of a group and the group has agreed that you speak for the other members.
- **Stick to your limits:** don't let yourself be manipulated or bullied. If you are being fair and reasonable, don't be afraid to raise your concerns at a higher level.
- **Remember the emotional and intellectual level of the person you are speaking to:** you may need to make allowances for people who are

very young or very old, who have just been through something very traumatic, or who have some difficulty that affects the way they relate to other people.

Asserting yourself can be difficult, especially if you have been raised in a culture where it is not right to complain or it is wrong to speak up to people in authority. It takes practice. Find someone who is good at being assertive and ask him or her to help you. As you become more confident and experienced, it will become easier and more natural for you to be assertive.

Assertiveness is a powerful leadership trait and developing it will be good for your grades, your career and your level of stress. However, always be careful to not become aggressive when you are being assertive.

BOUNDARIES

Let's be completely clear on boundaries: bad boundaries will get you into trouble, so learn good boundaries as a student and keep them during your nursing career. Nurses care intimately for people, and it is easy for boundaries to become blurred. You have an obligation – to yourself, to your patients and to your colleagues – to keep your boundaries clear.

What are good boundaries?

- Being attached enough to take care of someone, but not so attached you want to take them home with you
- Being able to say 'No' when it's appropriate
- Being able to separate your personal life from who you are as a nurse (this is tough for many people).

Some patients will really get to you. You'll want to help them, support them and take care of them. But you have to remember your role and respect that there are things you can't do:

- Don't give patients your personal contact details.
- Don't do things that are inappropriate (buying alcohol, etc.).
- Never, ever keep a 'secret'. What happens when the patient says 'Thanks for promising not to tell. I am going to kill myself tonight.'? If a patient ever says to you 'I'll tell you, but please don't tell anyone . . .', say 'I might need to tell someone else, so if it's really something no one else can know, I'd feel better if you didn't tell me.' Don't ever promise to keep a secret: if you find out once hearing the secret that you must share it, it puts you in a terrible position. If a patient won't tell you because you won't promise not to keep a secret, go to your mentor or a more senior member of staff.

● Just because you are the nurse doesn't mean all the patient's problems are your problems. You are there to take care of the patient, but you are one member of a team. If the patient has other problems – financial worries, relationship worries, etc. – don't let yourself be sucked into fixing things that you are neither trained nor equipped to cope with. Tell your mentor or another staff nurse what you know about the patient's problems.

● Don't tell too much about yourself. It's not appropriate to treat a patient like a friend – sharing information about your family and about your life outside work. It can also make it very difficult for patients to treat you like a nurse when they see you as a friend.

We can work so hard as nurses that we can forget that we don't have to be a nurse all the time. I remember letting it slip on one holiday that I was a nurse and I spent the rest of the week listening to people talk on and on about their constipation and their great-aunt's ear surgery!

You are probably very proud of being a nurse – and rightly so! But if you tell people you are a nurse, they may come to you and ask for help and advice. Or they might take advantage of your caring nature and bore you to death talking about things that no one else will listen to. They might even skip getting the help they really need and expect you to do things for them. As a student, you are not qualified to give advice – and anyway, don't you have enough to do already? Remember the limitations of being a student, and don't forget that if you don't take care of yourself then you won't be there to take care of anyone else.

At the beginning of this section I mentioned that bad boundaries are bad for your colleagues; here's an example

In America, I worked in a large team of community nurses. One day a nurse came in over an hour late for our meeting. She turned to the nurse on her left (I'll call her Sukie) and said angrily 'Look, you might think that doing Mrs King's shopping is OK when you do it, but then she expects me to do it!'

Sukie had a habit of being 'too good' to patients. Sukie did a little shopping, a little laundry, watered the plants . . . and that set up an expectation that we would all do the same. The patients didn't realize Sukie was doing 'extra'; they assumed it was part of the visiting nurse's role. Other nurses felt guilty when they said 'No' to these patients, and they were angry with Sukie as a result. Patients became angry when other nurses didn't do the same things that Sukie did.

Sukie was repeatedly passed over for promotion and struggled to get people to help her – they thought that if she had time to do extra then she had time to get her own work done. The situation was very unpleasant for everyone. And poor Sukie – all she was trying to do was help. She was an excellent nurse, very technically skilled; she just had very blurry boundaries. She didn't understand why everyone was so angry. She saw herself as a good nurse, felt isolated, and was very hurt when she didn't get promoted.

The moral of the story? Being 'too good' isn't too good.

COPING WITH STRESS

Stress, what a wonderful thing! Stress causes physiological responses that quicken our reflexes, help us learn and adapt, and get us out of trouble. However, if stress lasts too long we find ourselves getting tired, worn out and depressed. Our physiological coping skills start to backfire. We get 'stressed out'.

People have many different ways of dealing with stress. Some are negative:

- drinking, taking drugs, smoking
- food (eating too much or too little)
- becoming depressed
- withdrawal and isolation
- spending money
- being grouchy, irritable and aggressive.

Some people cope with stress in very positive ways:

- looking for solutions to the problems causing them stress
- exercising at the gym, going for a walk, taking up Tai Chi
- taking a break or a holiday
- going for counselling
- going out with friends and having a good time.

You are facing a very stressful time, from many different angles:

- you are financially stressed
- you are in a stressful profession
- you will become sleep deprived
- you will be learning a lot in a short period of time
- you will be exposed to the pain and suffering of people around you
- you will be worried about passing your course
- your important relationships could suffer
- you will find yourself juggling all kinds of priorities
- you will feel like you don't have any time
- responsibilities like housework, ironing, etc., could all feel overwhelming
- you will probably be working extra hours on top of your course
- you could feel bullied or harassed.

Depressed yet?

If you are, cheer up. It's never as bad as you are worried it could be. The whole point is to know what you are really up against. Let me give you an example.

My husband and I go on holiday in Greece. I love Greece – the sea, the food, the people, the history – it's wonderful. People in Greece have a very relaxed attitude about everything, and I find it very frustrating. When we go to Greece, and I get impatient because the waiter is busy talking to his friends and has been ignoring us for half an hour, or the bus is 20 minutes late, and I start clucking and carrying on, my (incredibly patient and sensible) husband says 'Don't you love being in the Mediterranean?'.

What he is intentionally reminding me is: I knew it was going to be like this, I can't change it, and if I keep getting frustrated the only person who will suffer is me (well, and him). We both know that I'll get stressed when those things happen – so he helps me recognize when it is happening.

Now, we plan ahead to prevent the stress. We don't go to a restaurant when we are starving; we go an hour before we really think we will want to eat. If we are in a hurry, we take a taxi instead of the bus. We plan to cope with the stress, and it helps us just enjoy our holiday.

You need to do the same with nursing:

- **Know what stresses you.** Some people are stressed by lateness or by having a lot to do, or even by having to ask other people for help. Know what your pet peeves are, and plan on how to work with them. Know how to prevent the stress from adding up.

- **Have time for yourself.** Many people find that spending good time with friends and family helps with stress. Taking a break, even when you are really busy, can help you calm down and focus on what needs to be done. Don't work yourself into a rut; take a day when you are not thinking about nursing, university, your assignments . . . you will go back refreshed and with a clear mind.

- **Don't get into a pattern of bad coping.** Coping with the ways you cope can be worse than the stress! If you cope by eating, drinking or going out, try to be aware that at some point you could go overboard and that too much of anything – even a good thing – can be harmful. Caffeine, chocolate, exercise and alcohol are good things in moderation, but could add to, rather than resolve, stress if used excessively.

- **Don't hide or procrastinate.** Don't stuff the 'final demand for payment notice' under the sofa. Don't call in sick because you can't face your mentor. Don't leave your assignment until the last minute because you feel you don't know what to do. All these put off stress momentarily, but make more stress in the end.

- **Accept that stress happens.** You will get stressed. Look at the context of that stress. Is it life-threatening? Is it worth allowing yourself to get worked up about? Is anyone going to die? A dear friend once said: 'The way I tell if I need to allow myself to get stressed over something is wondering if it would ever make the papers!'

- **Plan ahead for stress.** Give yourself permission to not be perfect. When you are going into something that you know makes you stressed, look at yourself honestly and tell yourself it's OK. If it happens, it happens. Believe it or not, it will help you keep control.

⬭ **Know who to go to for help.** If the stress really builds up, you could become depressed or have other physical problems. It's OK to seek help. Talk to your personal tutor, the student union advisor, your GP. If you start feeling as though you can't cope with anything, get help. It's normal to need help sometimes.

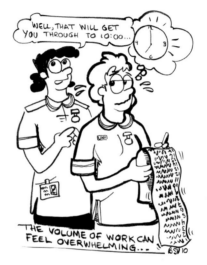

DELEGATION AND ORGANIZATION

These two concepts go hand in hand – delegation is sharing out your work with other people; organization is how you organize your day and your workload to get everything done in a timely way. If you organize your work, you can see what things you need to delegate. Does that make sense?

Let's talk about delegating things first. The NMC says it's essential that nurses learn to delegate appropriately. You can't be everywhere and do everything as a nurse. One of the most difficult things for a student nurse to get used to is delegating tasks to other people. Yes, believe it or not, you will need to start delegating as soon as you start placements.

⬭ You will need to prioritize; what can only be done by you, and what can others do safely and appropriately?

○ You will need to choose which tasks can wait until later and which must be done now.

○ You will need to delegate to qualified nurses what you as a student do not feel safe or prepared for, or feel is not within your scope.

Think for a minute about life before your nursing course. Imagine you are with a partner and you have two children. You do the washing up, laundry, cooking, cleaning, shopping, ironing, mending, gardening – the list goes on.

Now, you have all these responsibilities plus you have the added responsibilities of your academic work and your placements. No one else can do your course, so you know that you must always be the one to do the academic work – although you might ask someone else to get a book at the library for you or do something else that supports you.

Of the other tasks, you need to think, 'What can only I do?' You might decide that you must do the ironing and the shopping, but that the other tasks can go to your partner and your children. You still help out when you can, but you have certain responsibilities that come first. If an emergency should happen – one of your children is ill, for example – you can rearrange a bit, but there are always certain things that only you can do.

The same is true in nursing. There will be some tasks that only you as a nurse can do, some that you can always pass to someone else and others that you may need to do yourself or that you can delegate.

How do you decide what to delegate? Think of the following:

○ Legally, can only a qualified nurse do this?
○ According to trust policy, should only a qualified nurse do this?
○ Does this task require a nursing judgement or skilled intervention?
○ If I delegate it, does someone else have the appropriate training and knowledge to do it?
○ If it is delegated, how badly could things go if it went wrong?
○ Is there appropriate supervision and support for the person to whom I delegate this task?
○ Am I shirking by asking someone else to do it?
○ Is there anything to make me think it should not be delegated?
○ What is the best use of my time, for my patient's best interest?

The answers to these questions will help you decide what you can delegate and what you should do yourself.

Delegating isn't easy, but you will need to do it. It's especially hard as a student, but being able to delegate will show that you are thinking and behaving like a nurse.

When you delegate, you don't need to order people about. You can simply ask someone to help you. Be polite, but know what you really want. When you ask someone to help you, you need to remember:

- What, specifically, do I want the other person to do, and when does it need to be done by?
- do I want the other person to come back and tell me when it is done?
- do I need to give the other person any additional information about what I need done?

Be specific. 'Sara, can you please get Mrs Jones and Mr Bradley ready to go home? I'd like it done as soon as you have a chance; they need to be ready to go by 11.30' is better than 'Sara, get the patients washed up'!

Don't just send someone off to do something for you because you are too lazy to do it yourself! If you wind up with extra time, then go and help out other people. Then, *they* will help *you* when *you* are running late.

Delegating starts with knowing what you have ahead of you for the day. In handover, make a note of all the things that have to be accomplished. Organizing your day starts here.

Now think about a typical handover. You have eight patients; you have two HCAs working with you, although one of them is going home at 11 am; it is now 8 am and you have the following things to accomplish for your eight patients:

- bed baths and bed-making
- observations to be recorded
- medication rounds at 9 am
- three dressings
- a preoperative assessment
- two patients to be readied for discharge before lunch
- something to be picked up from the pharmacy for one of the patients being discharged.

Which things can only you do? Which things could someone else do safely without you? Do some things have to be done before others? Make a 'to do' list and prioritize the items in order of their importance – put what must be done first at the top of the list. Star the things that only you can do.

This is where you need to start thinking about organization. If you look at the things ahead of you at the start of your shift, you will be able to plan your day.

Organization starts in handover. Prepare for handover by writing down the names and bed numbers of the patients before you go into handover. Use a three- or four-colour pen and when things must be done, write them or circle them in another colour. Then you can see them easily and cross them off as they are done. Make your to-do list, triage and decide what needs to be done first, and then go out and get your work done – think about which things need to be done first, and do them first! Try to plan your work in a way that is considerate to other people. For example, if you wait to do the preoperative assessment until theatre calls for the patient, then someone is going to have to wait while you do it. If you do it right away, then the patient is already prepared and no one has to wait. Time-management skills are absolutely essential. As a student and as a nurse, you will always feel like you're juggling a lot of balls in the air at one time.

To be organized, you need to remember the following:

- What things are likely to interrupt me and how can I plan ahead for them?
- What things can wait until later?
- What things can I do to make things better for the next shift?
- What things are best done by someone else?

Think about the preoperative assessment in the list of things to accomplish above. You know that some time during the morning you will be interrupted by a phone call from theatre. If the patient is ready, that call will last 1 minute; if the patient isn't ready, you will have to explain and tell theatre when the patient will be ready, and when you go to do the assessment it will be more stressful because you are in a hurry. Doing the assessment first thing would save you phone time, an interruption and a lot of stress.

All during your work day new things will pop up and demand a place on your to-do list. If you always know which things can wait, you know where you can put new problems on the list. One way to know which things can wait is to 'triage' things on your list. Triage means sorting things out according to how urgent they are. I use an 'ABCD' system:

A   Absolutely must get done before other things
B   Better get done sooner rather than later
C   Can wait until later
D   Don't worry about it.

Absolutely must get done

These are the things, like getting the patient ready for theatre, which must be done before I can really concentrate on doing other things. Examples include a task that, if not done now, will mean someone has to interrupt my work later in order for it to be completed; and work that other people may be waiting for before they can carry on their own work – for me to find an X-ray, to give pain medication, etc.

Better get done sooner

These are the things that, although not life or death, are important and need to be done. Although no one will die if I leave them in bed an extra half an hour, it is unpleasant to be left stuck in bed – so I must get people up, washed and dressed after I have done all the things that can't wait. Sometimes you have to do some 'Better get done...' while waiting for opportunities to get 'Absolutely ......' tasks finished – for example, if you need a urine sample before a person goes to theatre (an 'Absolutely ...'), take the time to get the that person to the loo and get them washed up at the same time.

Can wait

These are the 'when you have a chance' things – things like going to the pharmacy to get something not needed until the afternoon. Some paperwork and administrative tasks are 'Can waits'. You just have to make sure they get done.

Don't worry

Some things are nice to do, but if you don't get them done it won't affect your patient care – things like tidying up the break room, putting together documents in advance for new admissions.

Sometimes things will go up in rank – for example, changing Mr Long's bed was down as a 'Can wait...' until his IV came out and blood went all over the bed, at which point it became an 'Absolutely ...'. Some things will go down in rank – for example, it was imperative that I give Mr Sullivan his preparation for endoscopy before 10 am, until they cancelled the procedure!

When I make a to-do list, I rank things according to my ABCD list. I don't really worry about Bs until all the As are done; I just keep going. I try not to take a break or get distracted until I have at least most (if not all) the 'Absolutely ...' tasks done. Although it isn't always realistic to do things that way, I try. If someone throws a new task my way, I rank it and it gets its place in my priorities. If I have a chance to get something else done easily while doing one task, I try to fit it in.

It takes time and practice to get used to organizing your work for a shift. Watch the way others do it. How does it feel to work with someone who isn't very organized? How does it feel when someone helps the shift go by smoothly? If you find someone who always seems to have things under control, ask how she organizes herself and learn from her.

ETHICS

Nurses work within a number of different ethical frameworks. Your university will let you know which specific model it will use during the ethics and law module you will take. Basically, ethics boils down into three main issues:

1. Do no harm/do good (non-maleficence/beneficence)
2. Trustworthiness/truth-telling and honesty/justice and fairness
3. Respect for personhood/respect for individual autonomy.

In some ethical models these will be teased out into more categories, but I have found it easier to think about them trimmed down to just these three.

Do no harm/do good (non-maleficence/beneficence)

The first cardinal rule of nursing, and of medicine, is *'Do no harm'*. As a nurse, you must look at the way your actions affect your patient. You must always consider: are my actions causing harm? What is the benefit for my patient? The patients and their families should never be worse off for knowing you! This doesn't mean that you won't, as a nurse, do things that cause discomfort, because we all know that it's inevitable that we will. It doesn't mean you won't do things that the patient doesn't like to have done. The key is that everything you do must ultimately be in the patient's best interest and not make anything any worse for them. 'Doing no harm' also means that you need to keep good boundaries and stay within the limitations and scope of your role as a student (and eventually as a nurse).

Trustworthiness/truth-telling and honesty/justice and fairness

Nursing is one of the most trusted professions in the world. Just because you are a nurse (or even a nursing student), people are going to make assumptions about you and your character. They are going to assume that you are a good and honest person. It's important for people to feel that those taking care of them and their families are people who they can trust. You have an obligation to uphold that trustworthiness. Part of the way you prove you are trustworthy is by being honest. The catch is, as a nurse, telling the truth isn't always as simple as just blurting out the most truthful answer you can think of. You have to find a way to tell the truth that *does no harm*. Don't ever lie to a patient. It's better to say 'I don't know' or 'I need to ask someone else to discuss this with you'. You also prove your trustworthiness by following the legal and professional codes for your practice, and behaving in a fair and just way.

Respect for personhood/respect for individual autonomy

As a nurse, you have an obligation to put aside any personal biases or prejudices. You have to see each of your patients and their family members as people who deserve the best care you can offer.

You must always remember that patients have the right to make decisions for themselves, even when those decisions are not the ones we as nurses or medical people would make for them. Some people may not have the capacity to make decisions for themselves: it is your obligation to do the best you can to make the decisions you believe in your heart would be the ones these patients would make for themselves if they were able to. Sometimes, we put a lot of pressure on people to make the decision we want them to make. To a limited extent, we can use our influence as carers to manipulate patients into doing what we think is best. But remember, there is a difference between someone saying 'Nurse, I don't want to do this . . . ' and a person saying 'No, I will *not* do this'. There is a difference between getting someone up when he or she has just had an operation and would rather stay in bed, and giving someone a medication or treatment that he or she doesn't want. Use your communication skills, educate your patients, and really listen to them. Even patients who have diminished capacity to make decisions – the elderly infirm, the mentally ill, the learning disabled, someone with an altered level of consciousness, or children – still have the right to be treated with respect, dignity and a regard for their personal beliefs, wishes and views. It's not always easy.

Ethics is not a clear-cut process. There is no easy way to make sure you are making the most ethical decision. There is no single ethical principle that is greater than, or more important than, the others. There are some ways you can work towards making ethically correct decisions:

- **Know yourself.** Do you have any prejudices, biases or strong beliefs that could cause conflict with your patients? For example, are you afraid of people of a different colour? Do you have strong religious beliefs that could make you feel that another religion is 'wrong' or 'bad'? Do you have strong pro-life or pro-choice beliefs? Could you take care of a prisoner who was convicted of rape or child molestation? It's OK to have strong beliefs; you just can't inflict your views on patients or their families and carers. You must be aware of those strong feelings that could cause conflict and develop self-awareness about how to prevent them from surfacing when you are working as a nurse. If you ever find yourself caring for someone and you can't get past feelings that are making you struggle to see the patient as a person worthy of respect, then let someone know and remove yourself from caring for that person. *Do no harm.*

- **Be a reflective practitioner.** Reflect on your experiences, look for the ethics in your decisions and actions. When you are making a decision, consciously look for the ethical elements and reflect later on what you needed to think about.

- **Try to see yourself and your actions from the patient's perspective.** Seeing yourself and your actions from outside yourself is essential for growth. It is a key element in critical thinking. When you see things you aren't comfortable with, make a plan for changing them. Don't worry about not being perfect – just look for places where you can learn and grow as a person and as a nurse.

- **Develop your own philosophy about nursing.** If you have your own philosophy about nursing, about yourself as a nurse and about the type of nursing you would like to do, it will be easier for you to make decisions. Yes, I am talking about actually sitting down and writing out a philosophy. Starting with 'I believe that nursing is . . . ' and 'I believe that as a nurse I . . . .'. Review your philosophy every so often. Carry it with you and, when you are frustrated, stressed or struggling to make a difficult decision, re-read it. If you outgrow your philosophy, update it. It will help keep you centred. It doesn't need to be an A4 page – just a couple of lines.

- **Ask someone else for help.** It's perfectly acceptable to go to a trusted colleague, teacher or mentor and say, 'I'm struggling with this . . . '. When you are faced with difficult or confusing situations, talk about them. You should never have to make decisions in isolation.

- **Be an advocate.** If you find yourself in a situation where someone has blatantly behaved in a way that you feel is unethical, it is your obligation to speak up. Always do the best you can to be an advocate for your patients and their rights. Refuse to do anything that you feel that you ethically cannot do, but support patients in making the decisions that they honestly believe are best for them.

A man is brought into the A&E haemorrhaging from trauma. He tells you that he is a Jehovah's Witness and does not believe it is right to receive blood. He understands the consequences of his decision. You know that without blood he will probably die. You disagree with him but you respect his decision. You don't give him blood. If someone else decides to give blood anyway, you have to decide if you are going to challenge his or her actions or not. It's not easy, no matter what you decide. If you were the patient, what would you want someone to do for you?

You will be asked to make some very difficult decisions as a nurse. You will be there when people receive difficult and painful news. You will be there when people are struggling to make incredibly difficult decisions. You must always remember that, as a nurse, you must put your personal beliefs and feelings aside so that you can be the nurse the patient needs you to be. It can be incredibly difficult to do.

I used to work on an ambulance. A young man who had been drinking had put his infant daughter in the car, but not in an appropriate car seat. He fell asleep at the wheel, crashed the car, and his daughter was very seriously injured. He was unhurt except for some cuts and bruises. The smell of alcohol was incredibly strong, and I am sure every person there – fire fighters, police, paramedics – felt certain that the man was to blame for his daughter's injuries. Despite being angry with him, we still had to treat him with respect and compassion. It was incredibly hard for us – it's a normal thing to feel protective and worried about a small child – but we all had to remember that behaving in any but the most professional way would be wrong. He had done enough harm to himself without us making it worse. All right, there wasn't a lot of small talk going on, but we took good care of him and comforted him the best we could. We put being good carers ahead of being judgemental. After we dropped him off at the hospital, we vented our frustration and anger about the situation to each other: he never saw anything from us but care and compassion. (The little girl recovered completely.)

It takes reflection, self-awareness and thoughtfulness to be a good nurse. Knowledge and understanding of ethics is a giant step towards this goal.

There may be times you will be called upon to justify your decisions as being ethically correct. If you can show that you have self-awareness, that you understand the ethical principles and that you put thought and consideration into the decisions you make, you will be able to trust that the decisions you make are good ones.

LEADERSHIP

Some students (and, sadly, some nurses) believe that a student nurse cannot be a leader. Many of the things we have discussed in this chapter are important parts of leadership. Leadership is about being the kind of person other people can rely upon and look up to. It's about making good decisions and being a good role model.

Many people think leadership is about being charismatic and having other people like and admire them. It can happen that way, but there is something much more important at stake than personal power and importance. Good leaders improve the NHS as a whole and, as a result, improve the care we give. Even just one student nurse can improve the NHS. The *NHS Plan* (DH 2000) clearly states that leadership is required at all levels – it *doesn't* say 'except students'. Surprised? If you as a student make a conscious decision to make things better, you *can* do it. How?

- Be politically well informed: know the trust, local and national policies, and the national initiatives, that relate to your area of nursing.
- Know theory as well as practice, relate the two and keep your practice based in evidence.
- Promote and role-model good practice (support good norms) and challenge bad practice.
- Challenge other people (with respect, of course) to follow good practice.
- Don't let your standards slide; don't fall into the 'It's not the right way but it's the way we do it here' trap.
- Look for opportunities to improve things. My mentor Fiona Malem told me 'Don't step over something – stop and fix it'. The person who finds the problem is the one who must take responsibility for it.
- Know the tools of your trade: assertiveness, coping with stress, good communication, delegation, time management and organization and ethics are important, along with your clinical skills and knowledge.
- Respect other people – colleagues, patients, families, carers, other professionals – for their abilities and contributions.
- Wash your hands and challenge other people to wash theirs.
- Be self-aware.
- Always try to see things from the patient's perspective.

These things might not seem like leadership activities, but they are. It will help to understand why if you understand norms. Norms are the values held by a group of people. They aren't written rules, but the 'way we do things'. The pressure that makes us obey norms is the approval or disapproval of other people.

Clinical governance (more about this later) is about making good decisions about resources, about human relations, and about following the guidelines and policies properly – that's the management side, running the business side of things. The way these business decisions get put into place, inspiring people to do things well, convincing people to take up the opportunities to learn – that's leadership. Without leaders, there is no one to show others what to do, no one to run the meetings, no one to investigate complaints. What is leadership that it is so important?

- ○ Leadership is about taking risks, but those risks have to be taken with an awareness of policy, evidence and people's needs. Its part intuition, part common sense, and part 'I hope this works!'
- ○ Leadership isn't management, but it considers the needs of managers. It helps meet organizational and strategic needs, while at the same time making progress to advance people's abilities and to meet their needs.
- ○ Leadership improves care and supports people in improving their ability to improve care (governance). It does this directly, when the leader says 'Do that', as well as indirectly by inspiring people to act as the leader would.
- ○ Leadership is about knowing where you are going so well that you can serve as a guide to others.
- ○ Leadership is balancing the need to complete tasks with the need to consider people, and treating people in a way that everyone feels that they have been treated best of all.

There's a lot more to leadership than this, but this is a good foundation. Don't start out in leadership trying to change the world – just make sure you do the best *you* personally can. You may be surprised and find that other people start to follow you – and that's the way leaders are made.

Consider the links between governance (see below), management and leadership. There are negative leaders – the gossips, the people who become caught up in traditional roles and power, the people who resist change even when evidence shows that change is needed. Standing up to these kinds of leaders is very intimidating, but it can be done simply by refusing to follow them. Refusing to follow is very, very powerful, so don't use it lightly.

If you think that being a leader means being powerful, you are right. There is a lot of power in having the approval of other people. If you are going into nursing because you like having power, well, put this book down and start looking for a different career. Still here? Oh good! Just remember, having power doesn't make you any *better* or *more important* than anyone else. More power just means the responsibility to use that power and influence wisely: a good leader is a servant. Think about what being a servant means – it means meeting needs, caring about others, doing what you need to do rather than always what you want, anticipating what others need, putting others first . . . . it's not easy. If you aren't prepared to serve, you aren't fit to lead.

As nurses, we are all equals with the same obligation to give the best care we are able to give at our level of education and experience. No one has the right to feel superior to anyone else. I don't know where the quote is from, but I have this written in the front of my diary:

> Those whom the gods would bring to their knees they first make proud.

It was a reminder to myself when I became a national-level advocate as a nursing student that I would be useless if I got too full of myself. That's another key element in leadership: just be yourself, don't try to act like less or pretend to be more.

When you see good leaders, you will know them. They are the people who inspire you, who give you confidence and who role-model the kind of nurse you want to be. They are the ones who help you and make you feel positive about the things you do. Watch them and learn from them: that's the best way to learn leadership. As you learn to be a leader, other people will be learning from you.

NORMS

Norms are the way we always do things. It's the habit we have, the routines that everyone in an environment expects and accepts. Let's look at the way norms work in clinical practice.

Imagine that in a particular hospital all the day shifts start at 7 am. On ward C2, everyone is very particular about being on time. The manager, the sisters, everyone is always there and ready to work, at 7 am sharp. You make a conscious effort to be there at 7 am too, because you know that everyone else does.

When you go to ward Z2, things aren't so strict. The ward manager gets there at 7.20 am, handover starts at 7.20 am, and nurses are still getting there at 7.10 and 7.15 am. How long do you think it would take before you started being late, too?

That's a norm. Although the rule says 'Be here at 7 am', the norm says 'We will not make a fuss if you are late'.

Now, imagine again that the ward manager from C2 takes over for the ward manager of Z2. She shows up on time. She says something to nurses who are late. People start showing up on time.

The manager's disapproval caused people to start to follow the rule again. If the manager isn't there for 3 weeks it could slip back into the old norm – unless leaders amongst the staff keep the new 'on-time' norm going. Eventually, the new norm will stick and people will adhere to it even if the manager isn't there.

Helping to maintain good norms is important in keeping the clinical area healthy. It's where you can practice assertiveness, and where you can work on leadership. If you know the right way to do things, and do the best you can to help make sure things are done that way, you are helping good norms to survive.

One point to remember: think about communication. Try to make your point about good practice without stabbing people with that point! You will need to use tact and diplomacy; 'Oi, what's wrong with you, we don't do it that way!!!' is not the way to promote good practice! The way you say things is important.

If you work in an area that has hoists but still uses lifting to move people, you are a leader when you say, 'I am not prepared to lift; I'll go and get the hoist'. You are encouraging other people to do the right thing. Just criticizing someone for not using the hoist isn't the right way.

Can you imagine the decrease in infections if everyone washed their hands properly? You as a student could be a leader, simply by making sure you wash your hands properly. Other people see you do it and it encourages and reminds them. You know how difficult it can be to do something when you don't see anyone else doing it – start a positive trend! That's leadership.

You can be a leader in another way, too. You can get involved in student advocacy, through your union, the student union, or as a student rep for your group. It's not easy and it can be stressful, but often there are opportunities to learn about leadership, genuinely help other people – and build up your CV.

Concerns about good leadership go from students to the very highest levels of nurses. Not long ago I was in a meeting with some very high-level nurses, and we discussed leadership, management and governance.

GOVERNANCE

Governance is a very important issue for nurses: it's the way we make sure that the right things are being done by the right people. You will hear about clinical governance, which is how we make absolutely sure the NHS is prepared and able to give the best, most appropriate care to the people who need that care. The concept of clinical governance as we have it now started with the 1998 paper *A First Class Service*; it was used as an umbrella under which a number of different initiatives and policies would flourish. Things like clinical audit, clinical effectiveness and risk management are concepts that stand alone, but are also huddled together in clinical governance. Everywhere you turn in the health service, you find clinical governance – it's the way we prove that we are doing things the way we should. But, because it's everywhere and in everything, it's difficult to define well.

According to the former Chief Medical Officer, Sir Liam Donaldson, clinical governance is:

> A system through which NHS organizations are accountable for continuously improving the quality of their services and safeguarding high standards of care, by creating an environment in which clinical excellence will flourish.

He also said:

> Above all, though, clinical governance is about the culture of NHS organizations. A culture where openness and participation are encouraged, where education and research are properly valued, where people learn from failures and blame is the exception rather than the rule, and where good practice and new approaches are freely shared and willingly received.

Clinical governance is a hugely important concept in the NHS; it is where we as an organization make absolutely certain we are doing the right things for the right reasons. Under clinical governance, you have issues like clinical effectiveness, which is closely related to evidence-based practice.

What else does it relate to? Well, according to the NHS's clinical governance website, it is also:

- patient, public and carer involvement (the things we do to work together, collaboratively and cooperatively with the public and other professionals)
- strategic capacity and capability (the planning we do for the service we deliver, the way we communicate as employees and as NHS organizations, and the overall arrangements we have to enforce, guide and review governance)
- risk management (infection control, assessing and managing risk, preventing bad things from happening)
- staff management and performance (recruiting, developing, and appraising staff)
- education, training and continuous professional development (training, professional development, an organizational approach to continuously raising staff to higher levels of competency)
- clinical effectiveness (clinical audit, research, assessing practices and procedures for effectiveness, and evidence-based practice)
- information management (computers, patient records, electronic staff records, intranet resources, policies, etc.)
- communication (how we work with those inside and outside the organization, from public to patients to providers and the way we keep people informed about what we do)
- leadership (from supervisor to chief executive, across administrative and clinical functions, the people who manage, guide and lead others)
- team-working (from teams made up of people to teams made up of organizations, getting communication flowing and sharing information on best practice)

There is no one element that is better or more important than others. They work together.

The site also states clearly that clinical governance is also:

- patient safety – not just saving money
- involving carers – it's not just for clinicians
- highest quality, accessible, all the time and everywhere – not just a bean-counting or box-ticking exercise
- lifelong learning and professional development
- collective responsibility – not just one person, not just one discipline
- involving everyone whenever possible – not a stand-alone function
- recognizing the positives – noticing achievement – not just a waste of time to satisfy bureaucracy
- common sense – not just paperwork.

As you can see, there are some big things involved in this and you cannot avoid it. Even as a student, you are part of clinical governance – and, because you are so new, because you are immersed in education, you have a chance to make a huge impact because you may well notice things that others do not. You will ask questions that others haven't. You have a huge role to play in clinical governance, both as a student who asks questions and as a professional in the making who is actively preparing to take up a professional role.

Governance includes things like Essence of Care, and Standards for Better Health (see below), Chartermark, NICE guidance, even alerts about problems with medication, drugs or diagnostics. Clinical governance is like air – it's all around us, even when we don't see it.

STANDARDS: ESSENCE OF CARE AND STANDARDS FOR BETTER HEALTH

There are some other tools you have that you might not even realize – the standards set out for healthcare.

Essence of Care is a set of factors and benchmarks that cover all fundamental aspects of care. (The term 'benchmark' comes from the jewellery trade, where metals were tested for purity and marked by the craftsman; this mark was proof that the metal had met the required standard – so a benchmark is something that proves a required standard has been met).

The factors focus on the most basic and fundamental areas: communication, personal hygiene, oral care, food and nutrition, privacy and dignity, record-keeping, safety, continence, pressure areas . . . very closely related to the activities of living. New factors are released when they need to be; most recently there has been a factor related to infection control and the patients' environment, and a factor related to pain management. The benchmarks are guidance for how we in clinical areas should help people meet their needs in the specific areas covered by the individual factors, through choice and respect for personal preferences, through providing health education and health promotion, and while maintaining safety, dignity, privacy and respect for the individual person.

When you are a student, your tutors give you guidance about what you need to do to pass: they tell you exactly what they require of you. Your Essential Skills Clusters come out and say 'This is the way it's done'. Essence of Care is the same: it is obvious through the benchmarks what should be done.

In Essence of Care, each factor is broken down into step-by-step bites, making sure that nothing is lost. Organizations are invited to look at the way they do things and raise their own benchmarks.

Standards for Better Health (S4BH) are a set of standards that organizations must prove they meet for their continued accreditation. They vary greatly, but focus on making sure that evidence is used in practice, that information about best practice is shared with the people who need it, and that patients are cared for in the manner that policy and clinical governance demands. The S4BH sets the foundation for many organizations' clinical governance programmes.

Summary

- Nursing relies on you being a healthy individual who can be assertive, have good boundaries and a strong ethical decision-making ability.
- You need to cope with your stress or it will affect your patient care.
- Leadership is possible at every level.
- Leaders are not more important or better– they are servants of the people they lead.
- Standards are in place so that we can make sure people are doing the right things.
- Making sure we do the right things, and that people have the right skills, is clinical governance.
- You can't do everything, so you have to delegate. Delegation doesn't take away your responsibility; it adds a responsibility to make sure the other person did things properly.

REFERENCES

Department of Health, 1998. A First Class Service. HMSO, London
Department of Health, 2000. The NHS Plan. HMSO, London

Website

You can find out more about clinical governance from the Department of Health website (www.dh.gov.uk/health/2011/09/clinical-governance).

7

Cracking the Code

❝ When I started, I felt like I would never understand what everyone was talking about. It made me feel so stupid! Now, I'm in my third year and I can usually figure out words on my own . . . ❞

Final-year nursing student

In this chapter

- Introduction to the language of nurses
- Nursing/medical jargon
- Medical terminology in general
- Anatomical positions and descriptions
- Word root basics
- Common suffixes and prefixes

INTRODUCTION TO THE LANGUAGE OF NURSES

Medical people speak a special language full of large words and strange abbreviations. We seem to love the jargon and tongue-twisting words. Why?

- They are part of the tradition of nursing and medicine
- It's like shorthand, where you can say something in one word that would take ten to explain normally
- It sets us apart from 'non-medical' people. It's like being in a special club with a secret code!

If a person told you that your patient was having a 'cabbage', what would you think? To a qualified nurse, a cabbage (CABG) is a type of heart surgery! A nurse talking to another nurse will use CABG instead of saying 'coronary artery bypass graft'.

A quick story . . . I was caring for a patient on a morning shift, and she was having heart bypass surgery (a CABG) that afternoon. From midnight the night before, she had been NBM (nothing by mouth) so she would have an empty stomach when she went to theatre (it reduces the risk of vomiting when under anaesthesia). I went to talk to her, asking how she felt. She said she was hungry but didn't mind because she was having cabbage that afternoon and she loved cabbage! The SHO (senior house officer) had told her she was having her CABG that afternoon, and she had misunderstood.

The moral of the story? Speak 'nurse-ese' to your colleagues, but plain English to your patients.

NURSING/MEDICAL JARGON

You will encounter a whole new world of words and meanings when you start your nursing course. Everyone who has been around for a while will use them, and will probably forget that you might not have a clue what they are talking about. If you have been a healthcare assistant (HCA) or worked in healthcare before, you are a step ahead. But whether you have been an HCA or are brand new to nursing, don't be afraid to ask what words and terms mean.

Here is a very brief list of new things you will be hearing about . . .

Word/phrase	Meaning
ADL/AL	Activities of (daily) living – things like washing, dressing, eating, sleeping, etc.
Bank (or agency)	Nurses working for an outside organization that places them in different areas to meet staffing needs.
Bed rest	The patient should stay in bed. He or she might be able to get up to the bed side to use a commode: you need to ask. 'Strict bed rest' means the patient must stay in bed at all times.
Bottle	A urinal – a bottle that men can pee in when they can't go to the loo.
Bowl	A basin that a person can wash in.
Clinical waste	Things that are yellow (such as bin bags) usually contain items soiled with blood or body fluids, or other yellow bags that have been used in patient care. This is clinical waste. Clinical waste is disposed of in a special way.
Commode chair	A chair with wheels that has a bed pan in it.
Consent	A 'consent' is a formal document through which the patient gives permission for a procedure or other treatment or activity.
DNR	Do not resuscitate – meaning that cardiopulmonary resuscitation (CPR) won't be done. It might be called other things, but it's basically a decision that nothing would be gained by trying to extend life through CPR. This doesn't mean other measures are not taken!
Domestics	The people who clean, often serve tea, etc. (good friends to have!).

Word/phrase	Meaning
Handover	When the present shift tells the new shift about the patients and what they need.
HCA/nurse	A person who works helping nurses and delivering care at a certain level under the supervision of an auxiliary nurse. Different places use different titles. Might also be clinical support worker, etc.
HO/SHO	House officer (HO)/senior house officer (SHO) – medical students and newly qualified doctors go through a progression of titles and jobs while they are being prepared for practice. House officers are newly graduated, senior house officers have been around a while. They are organized into teams under consultants.
IVI	Intravenous infusion.
Kidney basin	A kidney-shaped bowl. (In the USA, this is called an emesis basin; emesis means vomit.)
Mandatory training	Training that you are required to have at regular intervals, like yearly, by law – things like the fire lecture and manual handling.
NBM	Nil by mouth or nothing by mouth – the patient can't eat or drink anything at all.
Nursing grades	Previous grading system: A and B grades – mostly healthcare assistants; D grade – a basic staff nurse; E grade – more senior staff nurse; F grade – a sister; G grade – a sister/team leader; H – a manager. These gradings were replaced by Agenda for Change. Current system: Bands 1, 2, 3 and 4 – HCA/clinical support worker grades; Band 4 – relatively uncommon; Band 5 – entry level and basic level staff nurse; Band 6 – senior staff nurse or sister; Band 7 – senior nurse, sister, nurse specialist; Band 8 – manager, consultant or senior clinical nurse.
OBS	Observations – blood pressure, heart rate (rate, rhythm and quality); respiratory rate; temperature and oxygen saturation.
Off-duty	The time schedule. There are different shifts: 'earlies', 'lates', 'nights' and 'twilights'... there may be others. Ask the staff what times shifts start and end. Although you are supernumerary, you are on the off-duty so people can keep track of you and make sure you have the support you need.
Porters	People who transport patients to their appointments, tests, etc., and who also bring mail, supplies, etc., to areas.
Sectioned	When a person is 'sectioned', he or she can be held in the hospital against their will.
Sharps	Pointy things: needles, but also clinically contaminated items that could poke through a bin bag (glass tubes, etc.). These go into a sharps container.
Sister	A senior nurse. Male 'sisters' are called charge nurses.

Continued

Word/phrase	Meaning
Sluice	The ward's 'dirty room' – usually where you find bedpans, wash basins, soap, commodes, bins, a place to flush away body fluids, etc.
TTOs	To take out – medications that patients take home with them.

Note: Those nurses care for are called many things: patients, clients, service users, customers, individuals, users, etc. I like to call them 'people'. Some people seem to think that what you call them shows how much respect you have – that calling someone a patient demeans them, while calling them a service user shows you value them. I think people receiving care are more worried about the quality, responsiveness and accessibility of their care, and it doesn't matter what they are called as long as their needs are met in a way that minimizes stress, frustration and effort. Throughout this book I have tried to call them patients because, to me, those are people nurses care for. Call them what you will – but don't rely on whatever they are called to show them respect: you have to work for that.

The above list is not complete by any means, but I hope it will give you a bit of a head start.

Just a note...

Don't be ashamed of being new. If you really don't know what something means, ask. Don't just hope that no one will notice. Someone will! Yes, people might tease you a bit if you ask about something, but at least you are learning and anyone who criticizes you for learning isn't worth worrying about.

MEDICAL TERMINOLOGY IN GENERAL

Knowing some basics will help you to decipher medical terms. It is helpful to know that words in medicine are usually based on Latin or Greek words. There are three basic parts to most medical words: the prefix, the root and the suffix. Here's an example . . . 'Electrocardiogram'. For now, just try to identify the different sections.

In *electrocardiogram*, you can see three main parts: 'electro', 'cardio' and 'gram'.

- 'electro' means electrical
- 'cardio' means pertaining to the heart
- 'gram' means a measurement or test.

Put the meanings of the smaller words together, and you have 'an electrical test of the heart'.

If you understand basic roots, prefixes and suffixes, you will have a clue about what the bigger words mean. Understanding the medical words for the different parts of the body, and the way their arrangement is described, can help you understand anatomy and different procedures, tests and medical problems. It will make it easier for you to understand what is being said in reports and in notes, help you to communicate clearly with other professionals, and help you to explain things for your patients and their families.

Here's a funny thing – there is a type of communication problem called a 'mondegreen'. It comes from a part of a poem: 'For they have slain the Earl of Murray and laid him on the green . . .'. Some people thought it was saying 'For they have slain the Earl of Murray and Lady Mondegreen' (say it and it will make sense, honest), imagining this tragic figure who died alongside her brave Earl. It comes from hearing words blended together. Here are some others:

'The doctor told me I have prostrate trouble' . . . prostrate means lying down flat. The (consistently) male speaker isn't saying he can't lie down; he is saying his *prostate* (gland) isn't being quite as useful and user-friendly as it once was – but he doesn't know the word *prostate,* so he uses a word that sounds like it and that he recognizes. Another example of this is 'old-timer's disease' instead of Alzheimer's. Makes sense, right? Make sure people understand what you are saying. Make sure you understand. Otherwise, you too may find yourself alongside the ill-fated Earl of Murray . . . with *real* prostrate trouble!

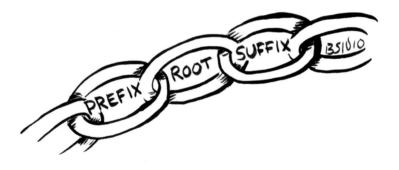

ANATOMICAL POSITIONS AND DESCRIPTIONS

There is a position known as the 'anatomical position'. Every description of the arrangement of the body is based on this position. Imagine someone facing you, standing on their tiptoes, with their arms by their sides with palms facing you. This is the 'anatomical position'.

Everything you can see from the front is 'anterior'. Everything you would need to look at from the back is 'posterior' or 'dorsal'. So, when you 'sit on your posterior', it quite literally means your back side!

Now, imagine a line cutting the person right in half, from the top of the head and the middle of the face; right through the centre of the body. That is the midline. Things close to the midline are 'medial', things away from the midline are 'lateral'.

'Superior' means top, or above, and 'inferior' means below or under. But the next terms are a bit more difficult:

- 'Abduction' means to take away from the midline of the body (to abduct means to take away)
- 'Adduction' means to bring in towards the midline (to add it to the body)
- 'Proximal' means closer
- 'Distal' means further away
- 'Flexion' is to bend a joint
- 'Extension' is to stretch the joint out again
- 'Transverse' means to go across
- 'Ascending' means to go up, 'descending' means to go down.

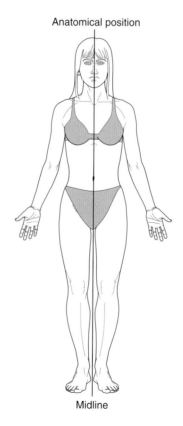

Anatomical position

Midline

These terms are used in descriptions, for example:

- 'The skin graft was taken from the posterior forearm' (the graft was taken from the back of her arm)
- 'She had a large medial laceration on her ankle' (the inside of her ankle had a large cut).

They are also used in the names of different parts of the body:

- Transverse colon
- Medial meniscus
- Adductor tendon.

It's always better when you can say 'the top one was 2×2 centimetres' instead of using big bulky words, but many other professionals will use the big words. Don't use them if you aren't comfortable with them, but you should at least know what they mean. So, try the following:

1. Which is more distal to the shoulder: the fingers or the elbow?
2. Which is medial (in the anatomical position): the little finger or the thumb?
3. If you drew a line across your belly, from hip to hip, would that line be transverse, ascending or descending?
4. When you lift your knee to go up a step, is it extension or flexion?

The answers:

1. The fingers, because they are further away from the shoulder, away from the centre of the body.
2. The little finger, because it is closer to the centre or midline of the body.
3. Transverse, because it goes across.
4. Flexion, because you are bending your knee.

WORD ROOT BASICS

Now, time to learn about roots, prefixes and suffixes. Try to see these as pieces of a puzzle, which when put together in the right order will give you the whole picture.

Root words are the basic words taken from (usually) either Latin or Greek. A list of the most common ones appears in Appendix 8. Some things will have more than one root word referring to them, like the kidneys, which can be referred to using the roots 'renal' or 'nephr'. It takes time to get used to them, but once you get used to hearing them they will make sense. After you have a root, you can use a suffix and/or a prefix to change the meaning.

COMMON SUFFIXES AND PREFIXES

Suffixes and prefixes are modifiers. Usually, the prefix modifies the root word and the suffix tells you something about the prefix and the root word. Here are some examples.

Anuria. 'A' means 'no' or 'absent'; 'uri' means 'urine'; and an 'a' at the end means 'a condition'. So 'anuria' means that the patient is not putting out any urine, for some reason.

Try another one:

Cholecystitis. 'Chole' means gall; 'cyst' is a bladder, so you know that the 'chole' part (the prefix) is telling you which bladder we are talking about; 'itis' at the end of a word means an inflammation. This word is telling you the person has an inflamed gall bladder. If it were just cystitis, that would mean an inflammation of the urinary bladder.

One more:

If *'chole'* means gall, and *'lith'* means stone, what is a cholelith? It's a gallstone!

Appendix 8 contains a list of root words, prefixes and suffixes. Some words won't follow the rules, but most will. Soon you will be amazing your friends and family with your difficult-to-pronounce new vocabulary. But remember, if you as a student nurse had to struggle to understand it, so will your patients. Speak in fancy medical talk to colleagues, but speak plainly and clearly when explaining things to patients and families. They won't be impressed by big words; they'll just be intimidated.

Safe and Accurate Administration of Medicines

> ❝ I trusted the nursing staff to care for my father. But, they failed him because they didn't do the right thing, and he suffered as a result. How can I ever trust them again, knowing how easy it was for them to let him down? ❞
>
> *Woman whose father's Parkinson's disease got much*
> *worse because of incorrect administration*

In this chapter

- Medication errors
- Safe and responsible administration of medication
- Nursing responsibilities
- Numeracy
- Dosage calculations
- Numeracy quiz
- References

MEDICATION ERRORS

The NPSA estimates that drug errors cost the NHS £750 million a year – more than £1500 for every nurse in practice in the NHS. That is only the financial cost; personal costs to both patients and professionals can't really be measured, but can be substantial.

As the person administering medication to the patient, ultimately it is up to the nurse to recognize potential concerns or identify errors before doing so. This can feel like an enormous task, but the NMC is clear in its expectation that every nurse knows the actions, purpose, usual dose/dose limits and method of administration, side effects, contraindications and nursing considerations for any drug she administers. Additionally, nurses have to know how to accurately calculate doses and rates, and convert weight and other measurements that can impact dosage, assessment or treatment. As it is impossible to look up every single drug before giving it, nurses also need to have some baseline knowledge about medications.

A medication error is defined as an error in the process of prescribing, dispensing, preparing, administering, monitoring or providing medicine advice, regardless of whether any harm has occurred. There are key ways in which nurses can help to reduce medication errors:

- Report all 'near misses' and medication errors, regardless of whether the patient is harmed, to ensure a learning experience
- Ensure drugs are administered to the correct patient by checking the wristband, and highlight antibiotic allergies on the wristband as well as the drug chart
- Check the name and dosage of the medicine to be administered against the prescription
- Do not check medicines and their dosages verbally in tandem with other staff to avoid talking each other through mistakes; do it separately
- Make drug administration 'protected time', and highlight this by wearing a bright tabard
- Don't be afraid to question other staff members, however senior, if you suspect something is not correct.

Giving medication is only a small part of nursing, but can be dangerous if not done correctly. Having good skills and awareness will protect your patients – and your career as a student and as a nurse.

SAFE AND RESPONSIBLE ADMINISTRATION OF MEDICATION

So, you know you have the right amount of the medication you want to give. Think back to the quote at the beginning of the chapter – there is more to medication administration than getting the dose right:

> The administration of medicines is an important aspect of the professional practice of persons whose names are on the Council's register. It is not solely a mechanistic task to be performed in strict compliance with the written prescription of a medical practitioner. It requires thought and the exercise of professional judgement . . .
>
> *NMC 2002, p. 3*

You will need, especially in the beginning of your career, to look things up every time you give them.

- Look things up in the *British National Formulary* (*BNF*) or get your own drug handbook (you can get your own copy of the *BNF* if you ask a chemist for a just-out-of-date one!). I like Mosby's *Nurse's Drug Handbook* from the US. It's not cheap, but it gives a lot of very useful information.
- Don't ever put something into a patient if you don't know what it is, what it does and what harm it could do. Your patients trust you to keep them safe.

- Always know the side effects and contraindications (reasons not to give) for any medication. If you aren't sure, don't give it.
- You can help yourself become more familiar by keeping a notebook and writing down medications, how they are given, what they do and why they are given.

As you gain experience you will become familiar with certain drugs and classes of drugs, and you won't need to look them up every time.

The seven rights

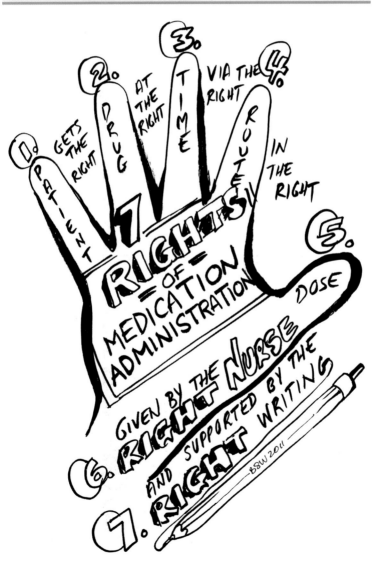

There are seven basic things you need to remember when giving a medication. If you follow the 'seven rights', you shouldn't ever make a medication error:

1. The right patient being given ...
2. the right medication in ...
3. the right dose by ...
4. the right route of administration at ...
5. the right time
6. supported by the right writing ... and
7. by the right nurse.

1. **The right patient:**

   – Have you correctly identified your patient beyond any doubt?

   – Is the patient properly positioned to take this medication?

   – Has the patient consented?

   – Does the patient understand what they are being given and why?

2. **The right medication:**

   – Is it appropriate for this patient to receive this medication? (Are there any contraindications?)

   – Does the reason the medication is being given make sense?

   – Is the patient allergic?

   – Are you sure this is the medication that has been ordered?

   – Is the medication within its 'use by' date?

   – Has the prescription been properly written by an authorized person?

   – Does the tablet or solution look cloudy, broken down or damaged? If so, double-check – how should it look?

   – Are you qualified to give this medication in this way?

   Make sure you don't crush or dissolve capsules or tablets without checking with the pharmacist. Don't mix liquid medications together without checking.

   Note: some types of controlled medication require two nurses to give them. Because you are not a nurse, you cannot be the 'second' nurse who checks a controlled drug.

3. **The right dose:**

   – Have you done (and had double-checked) any calculations and conversions?

   – Is the dose within the prescribing guidelines?

   – Is it in the right units?

   – How many tablets or units are you giving the patient? If it seems extreme, double-check.

4. **The right route of administration:**
    – Are you sure you are putting this in the place it is supposed to be? There have been cases of suppositories being given orally ... if you are not *certain*, double-check – don't assume!
    – Is this route appropriate for this medication and this patient?
    – Do you have patient consent to give this medication in this way?
    – Are you qualified to give medication by this route?

5. **The right time:**
    – For what time is the medication ordered?
    – Is this an appropriate time to give this medication? Will it keep the patient up all night, upset his or her stomach, or interact with other medications?
    – If the administration of the medication has been delayed, check before giving to make certain it is still OK to give it. Document that it was given late, with the reason and who told you it was still OK to give it.

6. **The right writing:**
    – Is this documented as it should be?
    – Are hypersensitivies/allergies noted?
    – Are the presence of any side effects and effects of the drug clearly noted?
    – Is it clear from the documentation that the drug either is or is not working?
    – If given 'as needed', is the assessment both before and after adminstration clear?

And ... lucky number 7 ...

7. **The right nurse:**
    Do you know enough about both this patient and this medication? Are you attentive to the side effects and the actions of this drug? Did you double-check correctly? Did you make sure there was no reason you should not give this drug?

Here are a few examples of things that can go wrong:

- The patient has a potent laxative ordered, in preparation for an investigation. The investigation is cancelled. Do you still give the laxative? After all, it's been ordered!
- Medication is ordered in pill form, but the patient is NBM (nil by mouth). Do you give the pills?
- The patient is allergic to penicillin, but flucloxacillin has been ordered. Do you give it?
- The patient gets digoxin 0.125 mg. The heart rate is 50. Do you give it?

◯ The patient is taking a medication in the morning but it says to give on an empty stomach at least 1 hour before food. Because of the timing of morning drug rounds and breakfast, the patient might miss breakfast every day. You look up the drug in the BNF and it says to give it at bedtime. What do you do?

Each of these examples requires the nurse to know more than what is written on the medication chart. You need to look up the medications and understand why they are being used.

Sometimes you might be asked to 'hide' medications in food or tell a patient a medication is one thing when it is another. This is called 'covert' administration. Although this might be considered necessary, there are legal and ethical issues that you must consider. Before giving medication covertly, speak to your mentor. If you are uncomfortable about giving a medication this way, you have a right to refuse.

As a student, you need to make sure that a qualified nurse supervises (stands there and watches) you giving medication, and that this nurse co-signs the medication chart (it is *your* obligation to get this co-signed). If you don't give a medication that is ordered, you should write up the reasons in the medication chart or in the patient's notes. You should also contact the prescriber if you discover a reason why you shouldn't give the medication.

If you find out that a drug has been prescribed improperly, don't just give it because you are a student and you think you don't have the right to challenge. The patient trusts you. You need to contact the prescriber. Perhaps there is a reason the drug has been prescribed to be given a certain way. If so, no harm comes by you questioning. If it was a mistake . . . well, wouldn't you rather know for sure before you give the medication? If you ever are unsure of the safety in giving a certain medication, don't give it.

You must never leave medications ungiven – not out on a table, not waiting for someone to give with a meal. If you don't see the patient swallow it (if it goes in the mouth, of course!) or take it, then it hasn't been given. Don't leave it out – someone else might get the medication; you can't be sure what happens.

NURSING RESPONSIBILITIES

As a student, there isn't much more you can do than be sure not to give the wrong drug; however, as a nurse you should know what the medication does, and do all of the following:

◯ If it has side effects, monitor for them

◯ Look to see if the drug is working – for example, if it's an antihypertensive, is the blood pressure better?

◯ Identify ways of helping the patient make the best use of the drug – for example, you shouldn't take tetracycline with milk

◯ Document what you learn

- Challenge those who do the wrong things; follow the rights and make sure others do too
- Look things up
- Ask doctors and pharmacists to help you understand what will help patients make the best use of drugs
- Check dosages in the *BNF* to make sure the dose you are administering is within the expected levels.

Special considerations

Drugs have special considerations; these help us make sure they give patients the most value. As a nurse you will need to be more careful, but, as a student, just try to learn and be more aware. For example:

- Parkinson's disease medications must be given spot on time or the person could seriously deteriorate.
- Always give medications for depression at the right time – those that are sedative in effect should be given at night; those that work by selectively suppressing serotonin reuptake, like venlafaxine (all the Prozac-related drugs), should be given in the morning.
- If you are giving pain medication, go back and find out if it worked.
- Give metformin with food, not because it needs food to work, but because it helps achieve the best insulin level to make use of the food.
- Just because something is prescribed three times a day doesn't mean it's 8-hourly. Think about what the drug does.

These are just some basics – as a nurse, you should do what you know your patient needs, by knowing what medications do and being sensible. Help your patients understand and properly use their medicines.

Summary

- Nurses must use good judgement when giving medication.
- Follow the 'seven rights' rule.
- Nurses should know as much as possible about the medications they are giving.
- Nurses, even students, have an obligation to question possible errors or mistakes in a prescription.
- Every nurse and student should have a copy of the NMC booklet *Guidelines for the Administration of Medicines*.
- Know what medications do, what their side effects are, and what patients need to do to make good use of them.

NUMERACY

> When I brought the 15 phials, my mentor said 'What are all those for?'
> I told her they were for the medication I was going to give, that I had
> added it up and this is how many I would need. She asked me if I thought
> that if a dose that big was needed, would the phials be so small? She also
> asked if I had looked up the dose in the *BNF*. She showed me how if I had
> given a child Oliver's age that much, I would have killed him 10 times over.
> The *BNF* even said how much to give, and if I had looked I would have
> known. I felt ashamed, stupid, and I am never going to make that kind of
> mistake again. How could I ever face life if my maths killed someone?
>
> *Children's student nurse*

> I can't do maths – I went into nursing to care for people, not count them . . .
>
> *New student nurse*

> NURSES WHO CAN'T ADD COST LIVES
>
> *Newspaper headline after research showing that failure*
> *in basic maths can have fatal consequences*

Numeracy is a key skill for nurses, not only because of giving medication but also because so many other things rely on measurements, scoring, conversions and the like. Even if you do not work in clinical areas, management or education, you will needs maths for finances and statistics, research, and so on. Every branch of nursing is the same in this – you *need* maths to be a competent nurse.

Although here I will do the best I can to give you a handy reference to jog your memory, you need to practise and become comfortable with conversions and calculations. I strongly suggest you get a book like *Nursing Calculations* by John Gatford and Nicole Phillips – it covers all the basics and will give you valuable practice.

It is true that there are those who are simply not good at maths; these people have to make absolutely certain that whatever they do, they make certain that their calculations and maths are correct. This might mean using a calculator, or it might even mean going to someone else.

The issue is that in any nursing skill, if you know you have a weakness, you are obliged to develop your skill so that your weakness doesn't hurt your patient and that you do everything in your power to prevent mistakes.

Some people say they *can't* do maths – I don't believe that's true. It might not come naturally, it may take a lot of work and you will probably feel frustrated, but you *can* learn. Even those with learning problems related to maths, such as the mathematical equivalent of dyslexia (dyscalculia, from which I suffer), can learn to both understand and carry out maths. If I can do it, you can. It took me ages but I am now competent enough to write about it in a book – so if you get discouraged, remember that it *can* be learned: I'm proof. If you really want to be a good nurse, you need maths.

Basic maths

Cheat sheet

Most common formula for drug calculations	$\dfrac{\text{What you need}}{\text{What you have}} \times$ What it's in = What you give

Conversions

cm/in	1 in = 2.54 cm	in $\times$ 2.54 = cm cm/2.54 = in
Celsius/Fahrenheit	$(C \times \tfrac{9}{5}) + 32 = F$	$(F - 32) \times \tfrac{5}{9} = C$
Liquid measure	1 ml = 1 cc	1 l = 1000 ml

Weight

kg/ lb	1 kg = 2.2 lb	kg $\times$ 2.2 = lb lb/2.2 = kg
stone/lb	1 stone = 14 pounds To convert stone to pounds: whole stone $\times$ 14 + 'remaining pounds' = pounds For example: 10 stone 3 lb = (10 stone $\times$ 14 lb) + 3 lb = 143 lb (*Remember to drop 'extra' pounds when multiplying* *stones $\times$ 14*)	
stone/kg	Convert to pounds first, and then convert pounds to kilograms	
Cheat factor:	Some measures to help you remember: 7 stone = 98 lb 8 stone = 112 lb (just over 50 kg; 110 lb = 50 kg) 16 stone = 224 lb (just over 100 kg; 220 lb = 100 kg)	
g/mg/mcg (µg)	1 g = 1000 mg	1 g = 1 000 000 mcg
mg/mcg (µg)	1 mg = 1000 mcg	1 mcg = 0.001 mg
Percentage	X% of Y = Y $\times$ ($\tfrac{X}{100}$) = percentage For example, to find 30% of 110: 110 $\times$ ($\tfrac{30}{100}$) = 33	

Other drug-related calculations

Concentration of solution	$\dfrac{\text{mg of drug} \times 1000}{\text{ml of solution}} = \text{mcg/ml}$	$\dfrac{\text{mg of drug}}{\text{ml of solution}} = \text{mg/ml}$
Infusion mg/kg/min	$\dfrac{\text{mg of drug}}{\text{ml of solution}} \times$ flow rate (ml/h)/60 minutes/weight (kg)	
	For mcg (µg) instead of mg, use: mg of drug $\times$ 1000	
Infusion rate in mg/ min	$\dfrac{\text{mg of drug} \times 1000 \text{ for mcg}}{\text{ml of solution}} \times$ Flow rate (ml/h)/60	
Infusion rate ml/h	ml of solution/60	

You have the cheat sheet, but without good basic maths skills, you won't be able to do the math needed. Here, we review basic maths skills. Look at the simple maths below: try these and see how you do. Some may seem very basic, but because everybody starts at a different place, and I don't want to judge anyone, I've started at the beginning. Try to do as many of these in your head as possible; only write them down or do them with paper if absolutely necessary.

How did you do?

1. $2 + 4 =$	11. $9 - 8 =$	21. $96/3 =$
2. $16 + 28 =$	12. $21 + 7 =$	22. $1152/32 =$
3. $23 + 99 + 23 =$	13. $43 + 6 =$	23. $400/25 =$
4. $247 + 389 =$	14. $32 + 4 + 7 =$	24. $900/15 =$
5. $398 + 878 + 37 =$	15. $323 + 89 =$	25. $3 \times 5 =$
6. $4378 + 8389 =$	16. $837 + 53 =$	26. $15 \times 4 =$
7. $12763 + 3237 + 233 =$	17. 15% of $9275 =$	27. $48 \times 36 =$
8. $4 + 6 + 6 + 2 + 6 + 9 =$	18. $33/11 =$	28. $480 \times 5 =$
9. $13 + 21 + 34 + 99 + 9 =$	19. $121/11 =$	29. $329 \times 235 =$
10. $37589 + 758 + 8397 =$	20. $156/12 =$	30. 30% of $2200 =$

Answers (don't peek!)

30. 660	20. 13	10. 46744
29. 77315	19. 11	9. 176
28. 2400	18. 3	8. 33
27. 1728	17. 1391.25	7. 16233
26. 60	16. 784	6. 12767
25. 15	15. 234	5. 1313
24. 60	14. 21	4. 636
23. 16	13. 37	3. 145
22. 36	12. 14	2. 44
21. 32	11. 1	1. 6

If you used paper for many of these, and you still got the right answers, you should be okay on the basics. If you had problems, think about where the problem existed:

1. If the problem existed in knowing *how* to get the right answer, you need some serious help, and need to let someone know right away. You will

need coursework. I can't help you if you don't know how to do the most basic maths. Go learn how the basics work, and come back. We'll wait here for you.

2. If the problem was that you knew how but had problems getting the numbers right, then we can work on that a little here. You will still need to get some extra help (you can go with the students from problem 1; I won't keep you long, so you can still catch up!) but I can give you some hints and tips before you go.

Hints and tips for basic maths

1. Always double-check your work. If the answers don't match, do it again and again until they do.
2. Memorize times tables. They will make your work much easier. Try to sing a song to make it easier to learn them (I still sing 3–6–9, 12–15–18, 21–24–27, and 30!) to remember the 3s). You can also get flashcards.
3. Practise as much as possible. Start to use maths whenever you can. Add up the bill in the shop or restaurant; figure out how many shoes and how many socks you have. Get used to not being afraid of maths.
4. Find a partner to study with – someone else who needs to work on maths.
5. Get some help – your study skills centre or learning resource centre will help you.
6. Remember that you are *not* stupid. If no one ever taught you the capital of New Hampshire, you aren't stupid if you don't know that it's lovely Concord: if you were never helped to learn maths, it's not your fault. Some people need more help than others, and that's OK.

DOSAGE CALCULATIONS

Basic numeracy is essential for nurses. If you are unclear about basic maths, your university should provide you with support to become more adept at the basics. If you know you have serious problems with basic calculations, ask your personal tutor, your library/learning resource centre or the student union about special courses to help you. The website www.bbc.co.uk/skillswise has good basic maths help – if you really struggle, talk to your university. Even if you are OK on the basics, keep a calculator handy and double-check your calculations with another nurse.

To measure, you need to make sure that everything is in the same units. Trying to figure out how many milligrams of something are in a kilogram isn't as easy as how many milligrams are in so many milligrams!

Here are some equivalencies:

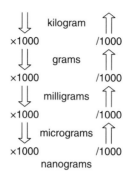

Remember that you must always use the same units of measure in nursing maths.

Try the following:

1.   Equivalents:
      a) 1 kilogram = _____ milligrams
      b) 1 gram = _____ milligrams
      c) 1 gram = _____ micrograms
      d) 1 kilogram = _____ grams
      e) 1 microgram = _____ nanograms.

2.   Convert:
      into milligrams
      a) 3 g, b) 12.3 g, c) 1.123 g, d) 500 g.
      into grams
      a) 1100 mg, b) 120 mg, c) 1776 mg, d) 500 mg.
      into milligrams
      a) 500 mcg, b) 5 mcg, c) 5000 mcg, d) 15000 mcg.

3.   Convert:
      a) 12503 mcg into grams (may be easier to go to milligrams then grams)
      b) 1500000 nanograms into grams
      c) 14 g into nanograms
      d) 1.23 kg into milligrams.

This book can't teach you all about conversions, but there is one small trick that will help you . . . a way to remember which way the decimal point moves in metric conversions. If you don't know how to convert in the metric system, it can be very confusing. This might help:

- To convert from a larger unit to a smaller one, the decimal point moves to the right.

- To convert from a smaller unit to a larger one, the decimal point moves left.
- You move the decimal point a number of places based on the difference between the units. It's usually three places.

It's very simple once you get used to it; you'll just need to practise.

> You know that a gram contains 1000 mg (1 g = 1000 mg). The difference between these two units, in zeros, is three places. So, you would move the decimal three places to the right to change grams into milligrams. If you have 250 g (250.000 g), you have 250 000 mg. If you have 250 mg, you have 0.250 g).

You also need to get comfortable with changing between metric and imperial measurements.

Weight

gram	g	1 g = 1000 mg
milligram	mg	1 mg = 1000 mcg
microgram	mcg (µg)	1 mcg = 0.001 mg
kilogram	kg	1 kg = 1000 g
		1 kg = 2.2 lb
pound	lb	1 lb = 16 oz
stone	st	1 st = 14 lb

Volume

litre	l	1 l = 1000 ml = 1000 cc
millilitre	ml	1 ml = 0.001 l = 1 cc
cubic centimetre	cc	1 cc = 1 ml = 0.001 l

Multiply litres by 1000 to get millilitres: 1.000 litre = 1000 millilitres.
By moving the decimal three places to the right, you went from litres to millilitres.

Length

metre	m	1 m = 100 cm = 1000 mm
centimetre	cm	1 cm = 10 mm = 0.01 m
millimetre	mm	1 mm = 0.1 cm = 0.001 m
inch	in	1 in = 2.5 cm

Multiply inches by 2.5 to get centimetres
Divide inches by 12 to get feet

Abbreviations are useful, but you should only abbreviate when it will be absolutely clear what you mean. And make sure you use good, clear handwriting. Print! Think what could happen if someone misunderstood you.

Only the most basic units are listed here: as you find others, write them down inside the back cover of this book. You will remember them more easily if you write them down yourself.

It takes practice to get conversions right, and you won't be alone if you feel a little confused about them. You will get used to it, and soon you will be an expert. Honest!

Formula for drug calculations

Calculations will be based on one of the units of measurement. The most common error is in converting one unit of measure to another.

$$\frac{\text{what you need}}{\text{what you have}} \times \text{what it's in} = \text{dose}$$

If you have the prescription 'give 1000 mg of paracetamol', and you have 250 mg, how can you use this formula to help you?

You need 1000 mg. You have 250 mg. 1000/250 = 4. What's it in? One tablet. So, 4 × 1 tablet = 4 tablets.

Lets try a harder one. You have 250 mg in 5 ml. You need 1250 mg. 1250/250 = 5. It's in 5 ml. 5 × 5 ml = 25 ml.

This formula is the most basic and common one in use. There are other formulae, but in general, this one is useful and will work well.

Sometimes a medication must be titrated (calculated based on an individual) to body weight or to body surface area (for example, a patient will receive 1 mg/kg of body weight). You always need to do the calculations using the same unit of measurement. This means there will be times you have to convert between units. If you are unsure of your conversions, have someone else double-check. It is good practice for any nurse to have someone double-check a calculation anyway!

Children's nurses will use special types of formulae and calculations. Children are not miniature adults; they are patients with very specific needs. Please get your information for these kinds of calculations from your mentor and from paediatric/children's nursing texts. I haven't put them here because I don't want you to take anything for granted when using them. The basics will still apply, but there are some very specific and important considerations you have to keep in mind; things too detailed for me to go into here.

In summary:

- Drug calculations can take many different forms
- You can't calculate a dosage until everything uses the same unit of measure

- The most likely place you will make a mistake is in converting from one unit of measure to another
- You should always have another nurse double-check your calculations.

Try this out . . .

You have 250-mg capsules (so your dose unit is a 250-mg capsule) and you need to give 750 mg.

(750 mg/250 mg) = 3 × 250-mg capsule

Dose: three 250-mg capsules.

You need to make sure you have the same unit of measurement or this formula won't work. The same formula works for other types of units. Try liquid . . .

You have heparin 1000 units in 5 ml. You need 5000 units. How much heparin do you give?

Dose: (5000 units/1000 units) × 5 ml

(5) × 5 ml

Dose = 25 ml.

What if it was the other way around . . . ?

You have 5000 units in 5 ml, but only need 1000 units?

Dose: (1000 units/5000 units) × 5 ml

Dose (1/5) × 5 ml

Dose = 1 ml.

What a useful formula this is! There are others, but personally I find that having just one and being good at it is what is best.

Numeracy Quiz

Although you can use a calculator, if you don't know what to put into the calculator, you will be useless.

In this section, there is a basic numeracy test. If you are not confident with all the exercises contained herein, you should look for a numeracy class. It is not enough to fake it: someone's life could rely on your ability to figure out the correct dose of a medication.

Just to be interesting, the first few problems will be word problems from practice. If you breeze through these, grab your trainers and go for a walk, you don't need this chapter!

Questions

1. Your patient is prescribed 150 mg of a medication. It comes in a 10-ml phial. The phial says '50 mg/ 5 ml'.

   a. How many milligrams are in 1 ml?
   b. How many ml are in the 150 mg dose?
   c. How many milligrams are in the bottle of 10 ml?
   d. Would you question giving this much of a medication? If so, why?

2. Your patient has insulin on a pump (these aren't real directions for an insulin pump, by the way). It has a list that says: Increase by 1 unit of insulin for each 3 whole millimols above 7. For every 2 units of insulin to be given, increase by 3 ml.

   a. The patient is on 4 units of insulin. The BM is 18. How much insulin should you increase the dose to? How many milliliters is that?
   b. What unit is blood glucose measured in? What is a 'normal' BM?
   c. Why do you need to be so careful when giving insulin?

3. Your patient weighs 15 st 10 lb. The doctor orders you to give 1 mg/kg of a medication. The phial says 10 mg/10 ml, and is 100 ml.

   a. How much does this patient weigh in kilos?
   b. How many milligrams would you give?
   c. How many milliliters is that?
   d. Is this a dose you would question?

4. You need to hang a litre of IV fluid. You are told to let it run in over 8 hours. The giving set allows 15 drops to 1 ml.

   a. How many milliliters an hour will this run?
   b. How many drops from that giving set will you need to set to make this run that fast?
   c. How much of this solution, as a percentage, should have gone in after 2 hours? After 4? After 6?
   d. How many milliliters should have gone in after 3 hours? After 6?

5. After 4 hours, the doctor says to slow the IV down to 1 litre in 12 hours.

   a. How much solution should be left?
   b. How many milliliters an hour is 1 litre over 12 hours?
   c. At 15 drops/ml, how fast should the drip rate be?
   d. If the original bag was hung at 11 am, what time will the new one be needed?

6. You have a phial with powder. It says to add 7 ml of normal saline, to make a solution of 2 g/10 ml.

   a. You are ordered to give 500 mg. How many milliliters do you give?
   b. How many millilitres are left in the phial?
   c. How many milligrams are left in the phial?

7. You have an order to give 2 mg of a medication, but you have only 0.625-mg tablets. How many do you give? There are no other tablets available.

8. You are ordered to give 750 mg, you have 250-mg tablets. How many do you give?

9. You are ordered to give 50 mg/stone. The person weighs 140 lb. How many milligrams do you give?

10. You are ordered to give 125 mcg. You have 0.250-mg tablets. How many do you give?

How did you do? These are similar to the kinds of problems you will need to solve as a nurse.

Answers

1.

a. Divide 50 mg by 5 ml to find out how many milligrams per milliliter. The '/' actually tells you to do that, as it's the symbol for 'divided by'. The bottle actually says '50 mg divided by 5 ml'. You have 10 mg/ml.

b. If 50 mg = 5 ml, then multiplying 50 by 3 to get 150 means having to multiply 5 ml by three, so you have 15 ml.

c. If 5 ml = 50 mg, then multiplying 5 ml by 2 to get 10 ml means you have to multiply 50 mg by two as well, getting 100 mg.

d. I might question it because it is using two phials, and most medications come within the dose that it is expected to use. Sometimes doses are bigger than the one phial, but it's a good hint that I should double-check.

2.

a. The directions are telling you to act if the BM is above 7. Now, you have to find out how much above 7 it is – so 18−7 = 11. You have to increase the insulin for every 3 whole millimols. There are 3 × 3 mmols, plus 2 left over. That gives an additional 3 units (one for each 3 whole millimols). If I need to give 3 ml for every 2 units of insulin, I have one dose of 2 units for which I can give 3 ml, but then I have 1 unit left. It's half of the '2 units = 2 ml' that's half of 2, so it's also half of 3 ml. I wind up with 3 ml (for the first 2 units) and then 1.5 ml (for the additional unit). I need to give 4.5 ml.

b. Blood glucose *in the UK* is measured in millimols per litre. A normal *fasting* glucose is usually between 4 and 7 mmol/l, although some say it's 4–6.5 mmol/l.

c. Insulin helps the body to use sugar as fuel. Without insulin, the sugar builds up and not only does it not go into cells as fuel but its presence (and lack of energy being released) also causes damage to fine blood vessels such as those in the eyes and kidneys. Too little insulin causes long-term damage across the body – we call the results neuropathy (nerve damage from neuro – nerve and pathy – disease) and vascular damage.

Too much insulin causes the sugar supply to be used up too quickly, which then leaves the person without fuel. Just like any machine with no fuel, the body can grind to a stop, called a coma. A patient can die from hypoglycaemia (low blood sugar); that is why you must give insulin carefully.

3.

a.   Each kilo weighs 2.2 lb. You have to convert stones into pounds (although you may have a table that converts stones into kilos, to practise maths it's good to convert). Try to develop easy ways of remembering key units and their conversion. For example, I know that 1 st = 14 lb; 10 st = 140 lb. I start with the 15 stone, and can figure out that 15 st = 10 st (140 lb) + 5 st (half of 10 st and half of 140 lb = 70 lb). That means that 15 st = 210 lb, plus the extra 10 lb, so the patient weighs 220 lb. Dividing by 2.2, I know that means the patient weighs 100 kg. (It's useful to remember: 220 lb = 100 kg. Now you also know that 15 st 10 lb also equals 100 kg).

b.   If the patient weights 100 kg, then at 1 mg/kg we would need to give 100 mg.

c.   If the phial is 10 mg/10 ml, and we need to give 100 mg, then we need to give 10 × 10 mg, so that also means 10 times whatever the volume is - so in this case, it would mean 10 times 10 ml.

d.   Probably not, as it is using one phial, but if I were not certain of the proper doses I would always look it up anyway.

4.

a.   I need to take 1000 ml (1 l) and divide by 8 to figure out how many litres an hour – so 125 ml/h.
     Just a note, when calculating IVs, you need to round it down to make it easier to figure out the drip rate (unless you are using a machine that does it for you). To run 1000 ml over 12 hours means roughly 80 ml/h, 6 hours is 150 ml/h, 4 hours is 250 ml/h.

b.   The giving set gives 15 drops per ml, and to set the drip rate I need to know how many milliliter in a minute. I know that 125 ml per hour divided by 60 min in an hour, rounded down, is 2 ml per minute. If each milliliter = 15 drops, then to multiply milliliter by 2, I also must multiply 15 by two, meaning that 2 ml = 30 drops per minute.
     Milliliters per hour/60 minutes (which is milliliters per minute) × drops per minute = drip rate.

c.   Each hour we are putting in one-eighth of the fluid, as we have divided it over 8 hours. After 2 hours, we will have put in $\frac{1}{8} \times 2 = \frac{2}{8} = \frac{1}{4} = 25\%$. You tell that by multiplying $\frac{1}{4}$ by 100 and seeing what you have left. In this case, $\frac{100}{4} = 25$. After 4 hours, it is $\frac{4}{8}$, which is $\frac{1}{2}$; $\frac{1}{2} \times 100$ (i.e. $\frac{100}{2}$) = 50%. 6 hours is $\frac{6}{8}$, or $\frac{3}{4}$; $\frac{3}{4} \times 100$ (i.e. $\frac{300}{4}$) = 75%.

d. At 125 ml/h, 3 hours × 125 = 375 ml.
At 125 ml/h, 6 hours × 125 = 750. Or, you could multiply
2 × 375 (volume infused in 3 hours).

5.

a. If 1000 ml was to go in over 8 hours, then over 4 hours 50%
should have gone in. 50% of 1000 is 500 ml – but, I would
need to check the bag to make sure.

b. 12 hours is 1000/12 = 83.3333, but 80 is an easier number
to use, and for the small difference that it makes (less than
40 ml over 12 hours) it makes the maths much easier.

c. 80 ml/h divided by 60 minutes = 80/60 = 1.333. That means
one, and a third. So, 15 drops × 1 = 15, plus ⅓ of 15 = 5 =
20 drops per minute.

d. The first 500 ml ran in over 4 hours, leaving the second 500 ml
to go in at 80 ml/h. 80 ml/h = 6 hours to give 480 ml, and the
last 20 ml will run in over 15 minutes. So, roughly (because
bags never have exactly 1000 ml in them), you will need a
new bag at 4 hours + 6 hours + 15 minutes = 10 hours
15 minutes, or 9:15 pm (or 21.15 h).

6.

a. 2 g = 2000 mg (always use the same units of measure
whenever possible).
(Dose desired) 500 mg/2000 mg (dose on hand) × 10 ml
(what it's in) = $^{500}/_{2000}$ = ¼ × 10 ml = 2.5 ml.

b. 10 ml − 2.5 ml = 7.5 ml.

c. 2000 mg − 500 mg = 1500 mg.

7.

This is a tricky one for two reasons. First, you can't evenly divide 2 mg
into 0.625-mg tablets. You get 3.2 tablets: how do you give 3.2 tablets?
You could give just 3, which is the closest you can get to the correct
dose. But the second problem is that this is obviously a very small dose
of something. Is it this small on purpose? Is 3 tablets a very high dose
of this?

If you look it up and it says that usual dosage is 0.625 to 1.250 mg,
then 2 mg is a high enough dose to want to check it out before giving
it. If it says 0.625 to 5 mg is the usual dose, then you would give the
3 tablets, and ask the doctor to rewrite the order (or call the pharmacy
and ask for other tablets).

8.

This is not a trick: try (dose required/dose on hand) × what it's in:

750 mg/250 mg × 1 (tablet) = 3 tablets

You might want to double-check in the *BNF* what the dosage should be.

9.

Doctors never order things to be titrated by stone, but this gives you a chance to use your conversion skills. You know that 14 lb = 1 st. You might notice that 14 × 10 = 140. You should just memorize that 140 lb = 10 st.

You should give 500 (i.e. 50 × 10) mg.

10.

Those of you who said something like 5 tablets – start over; whatever credit you built up is gone! Look at the units of measure. One is in micrograms, the other in milligrams. You have to have both in the same unit before you can do anything.

You need to either move the decimal three places to the right to go from milligrams to micrograms, or three decimal places to the left to go from micrograms to milligrams. To go from a smaller unit to a larger unit, move the decimal to the left; to go from a larger unit to a smaller, go right.

So, if we go right, turning micrograms into milligrams, we would have 0.125 mg. Try (dose required/dose on hand) × quantity: (0.250 mg/ 0.125 mg) × 1 (tablet) = 2 × tablets.

Does that sound like a high dose? Check it out if you are not sure.

How did you do overall? No one can tell you if your skills are enough; only you can decide if you have the competency required to be safe with maths. There are some basic rules that can help you:

1.   Always check with someone else when you are new, even if you are sure.
2.   Always think 'does this sound like a lot?' – especially when giving more than one of something.

3.   It takes 30 seconds to look something up, but months to explain why you didn't look it up. It does not save time to not check.

4.   Better to give the drug in a slightly different dose than to not give it at all. For example, if it says to give 500 mg of erythromycin, but all I have are 333-mg tablets, or if I have 500 mg of metformin tablets, but need 850 mg, I would call the pharmacy and ask: if other doses are not available, can I give the nearest dose I can find?

5.   Knowing what drugs do, what their usual dose is and what their potential effects are is mandated by your Code of Conduct. You cannot use the excuse 'I didn't know!' if something goes wrong.

6.   When dealing with children, infants, or the older person, remember that they are much more sensitive to drugs than any other group. Also, remember that whatever you give to a pregnant woman you give to her unborn child as well.

Summary

- You shouldn't abbreviate when writing units like milligrams and micrograms.
- You need to know how to convert units from the metric system into imperial measurements, and back again.
- You need reliable maths skills.

REFERENCES

Gatford, J., Phillips, N., 2002. Nursing calculations. Churchill Livingstone, Edinburgh.
NMC, 2002. Guidelines for the administration of medicines. NMC, London

Website

Contact the NMC and get their medicines management documents. Go to www.nmc-uk.org and download it for free.

Reading and Understanding Research

What this chapter is

- A primer to help you understand terminology
- A guide to help you tell the difference between qualitative and quantitative research
- Something to build your confidence
- Something to help you determine if the research you are reading is credible, or if there are weaknesses in it that mean it might not be right for practice without a better look
- Something to help you understand audit
- Something to help you plan the elements of research work.

What this chapter cannot be is a comprehensive guide to research – there are many 500-page textbooks that can't be that, so I can't hope to do it in a few paragraphs. What I can do, however, is help you until you take a research module, and demystify some of the terminology and phrases so you will have the confidence to tackle reading or critiquing research.

ADVERT: 6 OUT OF 10 DOGS PREFER NEW YUMMY SCRUMMIES OVER THEIR REGULAR FOOD!

This is an example of a research project being used to sway opinion. After reading this chapter, you will realize that what it *really* says is 'Out of the 10 dogs we could convince to try our dog treats, only 6 of them would eat them before they ate their own food, and the other 4 ignored them until their food was gone. And there were another 118 dogs who refused even to taste the yummy scrummies – so we will just tell you about those 10 . . .'

92% OF WOMEN ASKED SAID THAT GREY-BE-GONE WAS
THE BEST HAIR DYE EVER!

Would it matter if all of those women had just been given coupons for free Grey-be-Gone? How about if all the women asked *worked* for Grey-Be-Gone?

This chapter will help you look for things that could cast doubt on a paper, or that could show that a paper is credible and helpful. When it comes to *writing* research, well, that's a different book. Sorry! But, two out of three nurses asked said it would be okay – I did that research at lunch when I asked two of my friends what they thought.

In this chapter

- Why is research important to evidence-based practice?
- Research basics
- Reading research critically
- Applying research to practice
- The power of research
- Approaching research
- Writing a research proposal

WHY IS RESEARCH IMPORTANT TO EVIDENCE-BASED PRACTICE?

'OK', I hear you asking, 'why do I need to know this?' You need to be aware of current research, first, because the NMC requires nurses to perform what is called evidence-based practice – that is, nurses must base what they do on current research that shows that the approach/treatment actually works. Secondly, most nursing courses have a requirement that you are at least able to critique, if not write, a piece of research. Finally, because when you go for jobs beyond basic entry-level staff nurse, you will need to show that you are aware of current research and use it to inform your practice.

In addition, you know from Clinical Governance that you must seek the best way to do things, to make sure that the right things are being done in the right way by the right people. If you can't measure and compare ideas and suggestions, you can't tell if they are the right way or a better way to do something.

You will probably use research in three basic ways:

1. To inform your practice and the practice in your clinical environment
2. To prepare for exams and assignments (or interviews)
3. To produce an assignment about research!

There are two different types of research and these tell you different kinds of things:

1. Quantitative research is more reliable for things that need to be measurable. If the research is about the best wound-care product, it will tell you which wounds healed the fastest and had the lowest level of infection.
2. Qualitative research gives insight into thoughts, feelings and experiences. For example, when considering the question 'How do patients feel about larval therapy (maggots)?', it is less important to know that x% said they would never try it than to know *why* they didn't want to try it. Then, as a nurse, you could use the research to help you find a way to help *your* patients.

In evidence-based practice, you should be constantly asking yourself: 'Is this the best way'? Research can help you answer that question. It's not as simple as finding one paper that says 'Yes, it is the right way'; you have to decide if you are going to believe what the research has to say.

Don't *ever* take for granted *anything* you read. Just because it's published in a book doesn't mean it's absolutely true! It's up to you to decide what you can believe in and what you can't. Evidence-based practice doesn't mean accepting whatever falls out of the first book you get your hands on; it means knowing that the evidence you are using is credible and reliable. Even as a nursing student, you have to be prepared to critically analyze your evidence base.

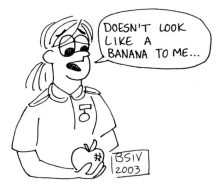

RESEARCH BASICS

Let's compare the two basic types of research:

Qualitative	Quantitative
Sample size	
Usually small (10–20)	Usually large (1001)
Each person gives a lot of data	Each person gives a smaller, more specific amount of data
Reported using	
Narration and excerpts; the data are usually narrative	Statistics, tables, charts; the data are measurable
Gathered	
Talking, interviewing, through group discussions and open-ended questions	Questionnaires with set answers, reviews of data and demographical information, measurements
Replicable?	
Not specifically	Yes

Now let's look at an example:

Question	Qualitative research	Quantitative research
What kinds of people become nurses?	Caring people, thoughtful people, people with strong backs, people who like dealing with other people, women	50% of nursing students are over the age of 30; 70% are women. Of 2000 people questioned, 42% said nurses were caring people*

* These results are made up just to give an example.

See the difference? Knowing the type of research lets you know what kind of data the research was based on, and what kinds of evidence the research will give you.

Clinical Audit

Clinical audit is a process by which we listen to what is happening in practice (that's what audit means – to listen) and we make changes based on how it should look and sound. We put actions in place, and go back and see if those actions are effective. Although not strictly research, you can learn a lot and make real improvements.

Types of clinical audit include:

- **Service evaluations.** These involve looking at a given service and asking: Does this work? How does it work? For whom does it work? Should it do anything differently? Does it do everything it should?
- **Audit against standards.** If the NICE guidance says every person should have a VTE (venous thromboembolism) risk assessment when admitted to hospital, do they?
- **Audit against action plans.** If you have advised staff that they now need to put their printed name and role with their signature, have they?
- **Patient satisfaction.** Although not strictly audit, listening to and involving patients is key, so asking them what they think of the service they receive is a strong element of research and audit – but cannot stand alone, and neither can staff satisfaction surveys.
- **National audits.** There are national audits in specialist areas such as sickle cell, continence, dementia, bone health, etc. National bodies gather data from all over and make a large report on services and outcomes.

We can identify if it's a type of research or audit from the research statement:

1. This research plans to explore the experiences of pre-registration students during their first clinical placement.
2. This research will determine the average class size of pre-registration nursing students in England.
3. This research will discuss the sizes of hydrocolloid dressings available to independent nurse prescribers.
4. This research will review if changes to the documentation template for nursing assessment have improved the quality of the nurse admission.
5. Review of the impact of the diabetes service, including uptake by various cultural groups, ages and levels of clinical need.

Number (1) is qualitative research – it is looking at feelings and experiences; (2) is quantitative research – it is looking at data that can be measured; and (3) is also quantitative research, even though it says it will 'discuss', because it is looking at data that can be measured. Number (4) is an excellent clinical audit topic – although it could also become a mixed qualitative and quantitative research paper; (5) is a service review. To understand research, you also need to know how to dissect a research paper.

READING RESEARCH CRITICALLY

Although research articles can be laid out in many different formats, they almost always contain the same sections. As you read through these sections you will need to ask yourself certain questions. Remember: your goal is to determine if this research is appropriate for you to use as evidence to base your decisions and your practice on. You need to think critically!

Author

When you are looking for research, the first thing you will see is the name of the author, the title of the article and the journal where it is published. These things start to tell you about the nature of the research. First, you need to establish that the author is a credible person, who has the background and education to write/research a paper of this type. Ask yourself:

- Does the author have academic and/or research credentials?
- If you do a search for the author, what other kinds of papers and research come up?
- Where does the author work? What is his or her expertise?

Title

This should sum up what the research is about. The title should give a clear indication of the nature of the paper:

- What expectations does the title give you about the nature and content of the article?
- Is it clear and specific?
- Does it make sense?
- Does it tell you how this is different than the 1000 other papers of a similar name?

Go back to the title after you have read the paper and compare it to what you *thought* it meant before you read the paper. Is there a difference?

Where is the article? The name of the journal

Some journals have a reputation for being very academic and reliable. Others may be seen as less academic and more 'fluffy'. You need to think about the kind of journal you found the research in:

- Is this a credible journal (e.g. was there an article in it about how to cut the toenails of the Beast of Bodmin)?
- What is the journal's audience?
- Is it the journal of a particular group or organization, and could that present a bias?

If an article on the healing properties of honey appears in a journal published by the Society of Beekeepers, you might worry that it could be biased because the people publishing the journal have something to gain by encouraging you think that honey is good. The same article published in the Journal of Advanced Wound Care would have more credibility, because the people publishing it have nothing to gain by your buying honey. In the same light, an article about building beehives published in the *Wound Care Journal* wouldn't be taken seriously by beekeepers (assuming they ever see it!).

Abstract and key words

The abstract and key words help you get a general idea of what the article is about. The key words are listed to help you find the article when you do an electronic search. If you want to search for similar articles to the one you have just read, search using the key words.

Read the abstract before you read the paper. Then, after you've read the paper, compare what the research said with what the abstract promised it would say. Do they match? Did the abstract leave anything important out?

Introduction

The introduction introduces the research question and sets the scene for what will come. You should ask yourself:

- Why did someone feel this was important to research?
- How and why is this relevant to nursing practice?
- Is the need for this research supported?
- Is the research question sensible?
- Is the research question something that is answerable?
- Is this the right kind of research for this kind of question?

Literature review

The introduction often contains a literature review. Doing a literature review is a real art. In it you will find other information and research available about the topic under investigation. To learn to do a literature review, you will need to read a book about research (there are some suggestions in the Useful Books, Journals and Other Resources section at the end of this book). To review the literature, you need to ask yourself:

- Is this new research a replication of old research?
- What has changed since previous research was done on this issue?
- Are the sources cited in the literature review accessible and credible?

- If there are other sources (which you would know about because you did a search), why haven't they been used?
- Is the literature review biased in any way?

You will need to look at the different sources listed in the literature review in the same way you are looking at the piece of literature in which they are contained – that is, critically. If the literature review is based on shoddy and unreliable sources, it could affect the credibility of the research overall.

Method

This area talks about how the research is done. It should be broken down into more specific subsections. If it isn't, you might want to question why. The next few headings can all come under 'Method'.

Sample

This explains who participated in the research, how they were found and why they were chosen. You need to look critically at the sample size and selection:

- Who was chosen to participate? Why?
- Were these appropriate sources?
- Is the method of choosing the sample appropriate?
- How long ago was this done? Has anything significant changed since then?
- Is confidentiality maintained?
- Is the sample size too big or too small?
- Does the size and type of sample match the type of research being done?

Also, think: if you were a member of the sample, would you feel that the research adequately represented what you said and did?

Ethical issues

What ethical considerations are there, and how are they addressed? Remember your ethical principles. Research must be presented accurately, but participants have a right to confidentiality.

To protect research participants and to ensure quality research, researchers must bring their proposals to an 'ethics committee'. This committee will look at the research question, the planned sample and methodology, and the ways that the research plans on resolving any ethical issues raised during or by the research. This includes protecting the confidentiality of the participants:

- Did the author get ethical approval for this work?
- Did participants give consent?

○ How did the author find participants?

○ Were there any special considerations for the participants?

○ How is participant confidentiality protected?

○ Did the author have permission, from organizations, workplaces, etc., to do this research?

○ Are there any issues raised as a result of this research that have ethical considerations? For example, if the research was into the use of a particular medication and it was found early on that a particular dose of this medication was dangerous, did research continue using that dose or stop it?

Data collection

How were the data collected? What method of collection was used, and how did it work? Data can be collected in many different ways, using 'tools'. Some tools could be interviews, questionnaires or focus groups. This section should explain the tool that the researcher used. You could then look that tool up in a research text to find out if the researcher used and applied it properly:

○ Is this an appropriate way to collect these data?

○ Is the tool reliable?

○ Is the tool used properly?

○ Does the research type support the tool? For example, if this is quantitative research and a survey was used, did it really produce the right kind of data for that method?

Using an inappropriate tool can skew the data, so it is important that you are critical about the way the data were collected.

Validity/reliability/rigour

'Validity' and 'reliability' are terms used to discuss how credible the data are. Data collected for quantitative research are held to a very specific standard: researchers must prove that the numbers and statistics being presented could be replicated in another study. This proves that the information they are presenting is accurate and correct. Qualitative research doesn't have to prove it can be replicated; in fact, it is expected that qualitative research could not be specifically repeated. Qualitative researchers prove their data are accurate and correct by showing they were rigorously using the correct methods and took every possible opportunity to remove any researcher bias.

To determine if the research is reliable, you need to ask:

○ Do the data make sense?

○ If the data are based on any other sources, are they credible sources?

○ How has the reliability of the data been tested?

○ Could this study be replicated with comparable results?

○ Are there any assumptions being made?

Results/discussion

This is where the researcher tells you the results of the study. The researcher will refer back to statistics and information from the sections that have come before. To make an analysis of this section, you need to ask:

○ Does it make sense?

○ Is it useful?

○ Does it match with the title and the abstract?

○ How do these findings compare with the literature review? Is there anything significant in literature *not* included in the review?

○ Are the statistics reported accurately? Do they match?

○ Are findings reported in a way that appears biased?

○ Do the tables, graphs and statistics actually tell you anything?

○ Do the data-collection methods and the data that are presented match?

Compare what you find in the summary with what the title, abstract and introduction said. Does it all go together or does it seem like they are talking about different things?

Summary

The summary wraps up the research. It gives conclusions, which may include recommendations or suggestions. It may suggest areas for further study. It might highlight any particular problems or obstacles the researcher encountered. It should answer the research question. Ask yourself:

○ Does it make sense?

○ Has the question been answered?

○ Does it offer ideas for the way forward or to change/reinforce practice?

○ Are there areas of future work that should be done as a result of this research?

After the summary come the parts that compare to the movie credits – you know, the parts that scroll by too fast and that no one really looks at anyway because they are trying to dig the popcorn out of their shoes as they leave the cinema. Well, it pays to look at these areas when you are critiquing research.

Acknowledgements

This section tells you if the research was sponsored or done on behalf of any-one else. You can find out if there could have been a bias in the research. Which would you find more credible: research that has been sponsored by the makers of product X about how product X is the best wound dressing, or the same research offered by the tissue viability department of a teaching hospital? So ask yourself:

- Did the supporter(s) of the research have a vested interest in its outcome?

Referencing

When checking the references from the text of the article, consider the following:

- Were any references left out?
- Does the author often reference him- or herself?
- Are these the sources that you would have used?
- How old are the sources? Are they outdated?
- Are they obscure, difficult-to-find sources?

If you are worried that the article could be biased, get hold of a couple of the sources. Does the way they present their data match the way they have been presented in your research?

Once you decide that the research is valid – that it is reputable and that it makes useful recommendations – you will want to find ways of applying it to your practice.

APPLYING RESEARCH TO PRACTICE

There are three key ways you apply research to practice:

1. By using it in your papers and, by doing this, getting to know what is right and what is not.
2. By reading new pieces of research and finding out that there is some-thing you should do differently.
3. By doing research and then directly or indirectly proving something is not as it should be, or that there is a better way to do something.

As a pre-registration student, you are unlikely to be doing much hard research (and a deep sigh of relief I can hear, too). But it is certain that you will be read-ing research for papers and as part of learning about nursing and care.

THE POWER OF RESEARCH

If you were to read an article that said drinking milk is proven to be bad for you if you are taking a certain antihypertensive (high blood pressure tablet), and you knew that many people in your clinical area were taking that tablet, what would you do?

You could:

- ignore it and hope someone else reads the research
- bring the research in and show it to everyone
- start asking people if they have ever heard of the research
- tell all the patients on that tablet about the research
- commission a new research project to prove the same thing.

Before you decide, let's reflect for a moment on the power of research.

The Editor of *The Lancet* had been criticized by a writer at *The Times* (18 June 2005) for 'scaremongering' by publishing questionable research. *The Times* said as a credible and renowned journal, *The Lancet* had a requirement to make absolutely sure that everything it published was absolutely correct – but in hindsight there were some problems with some of the research *The Lancet* had published. But *The Lancet* being a pillar of the medical community that it is, people were inclined to believe anything said in it as truth because if it wasn't, then it wouldn't be in *The Lancet*. Even when it might have been wrong, it was still believed.

The Editor said he did the best he could, and over time it was proven that some of the research wasn't quite as shaky as it seemed. But the damage was done. That's what happens in research: credibility and reliability are crucial, because without them it is difficult to believe and have faith in the results.

The dilemma (an ethical dilemma is a problem with no easy solution) for the Editor is – should he publish exciting but potentially flawed, incorrect or unbalanced research, or should he wait for absolute proof and maybe someone who might have benefited doesn't get the help they need? Would it be better to hide research that says something is very bad until there is more than one study, or is one enough? Would he be criticized for waiting for proof? Or for publishing incorrect research? Or would he be seen as a hero for breaking the one study that showed how bad something really, really was? He has to weigh the choices, knowing that sometimes there is no right answer.

See the huge responsibility research puts on us? Now, remembering all that, go back to the scenario about the milk and the antihypertensives.

Could you:

- ignore it and hope someone else reads the research? No; once you know research exists, you have to bring it to someone's attention.
- bring the research in and show it to everyone? Yes, you could do that.
- start asking people if they have ever heard of the research? You could do that, too.

- tell all the patients on that tablet about the research? Based on one study, would you want to worry and upset patients?
- commission a new research project to prove the same thing. If you could it might be good, but can you?

It makes a difference what the end result is – if the end result is that taking milk with that antihypertensive gives you wind, no one is really going to be too worried; if it makes you more susceptible to a fatal heart attack, you might worry more.

The application of research

There are two main ways to apply research:

1. macro – to a whole service, whole organization or whole company
2. micro – to one unit, one practice, one nurse.

Much of the research you will read – the articles in the *Nursing Standard*, for example – will apply just to you and other nurses like you. It will be evidence about how to perform better, how to do things more efficiently or in a way that is better for the patient.

NICE puts out guidance all the time that is meant for both macro and micro application – it says: 'This is how the entire organization should act as a result, and this is what the individual practitioner should do.'

So, that's a good hint – in research, the most important application is how you personally do things. If you read research that explains the best way to take a blood pressure, then you should take a blood pressure that way, and you should make sure that anyone you delegate to take a blood pressure does it that way too. You should bring it in and show your manager – but if she chooses not to have everyone do it that way, well, as a nurse who is more senior, she can choose not to – but you can also choose to ask her why!

Another way to personally apply research is to be aware of the research when you use policy, guidelines, care plans, etc., in your clinical area – if you know, for example, that research says you need to wash your hands before you take a BM (blood glucose machine) sample, and the policy doesn't say to wash hands, then you should challenge the policy.

If there is no care plan that tells you to turn someone every 2 hours when they are in bed, and you have proof that turning someone every 2 hours is something you should do, then you should bring that research to the attention of the person who provides that document – and start documenting that you turn people every 2 hours, whether the care plans ask you to or not.

Basically, research is there to tell you this: 'We looked at everything, and we found out that the best way to do this is to . . .'. There will be research that contradicts other research, or research so full of gobbledygook that you won't understand a single word. What is important for you as a student is that you take the time to get familiar with research, and that you start to allow research to teach you how to be the best nurse possible. In the beginning you will need help in applying research, but in time it gets easier.

You know why I am telling you about research? Because I did research and it told me that students are worried about research and evidence-based practice – so I decided to tell you. Isn't research useful?

APPROACHING RESEARCH

When reading research, read the title, abstract, discussion and summary first. If the material is not relevant or useful to you, drop it. This will save you from wading through paragraphs of methodology and design only to find out that the material doesn't really apply to you.

Some hints for better grades:

- *Do research on your research*. Look–up the author in CINAHL, Ovid, BNI or even just in the library. What else has he or she written? Does this add to or detract away from his or her credibility? Can you use anything else this researcher has written in your critique or support of this piece of work?
- *Do your own literature search*. Look-up related articles from the key words listed. Did the researcher leave out things that look to you as though they should have been included? Is there any newer research than this piece? If you need help learning to do literature searches, look in the library or learning resource centre. There should be information and probably even a friendly person who can help you learn to access the different resources available. Get a good study skills book (like the one by Maslin-Prothero, which is listed in the Useful Books, Journals and Other Resources chapter at the end of this book) to help you.
- *Think about your practice*. Is there something you wish the research had given you, but didn't? Is the information it gave you practical?
- *Be a critical reader*. Don't automatically believe everything someone says just because they wrote it down and researched it. Being a good nurse means thinking critically.

If you want to learn to *do* research, some of the books in the Useful Books, Journals and Other Resources section at the end of this book can help. But even if you never plan to research anything, it is essential that you can read research critically. Your ability to base your practice in evidence means you need to be able to tell good evidence from bad.

WRITING A RESEARCH PROPOSAL

When you want to do research, you have to develop a proposal and show how you will undertake the research. You then submit the proposal to an ethics or research committee, which makes sure it meets all the criteria (hint: find out the criteria used . . .) and that it is a valid topic. The committee will do one of three things:

- say 'go ahead'
- say 'uhm, can we talk to you about a few things first?'
- say 'No!'

The committee will send written feedback. Needless to say, such a detailed review takes time so deadlines are very tight.

To be blunt, a good proposal will mean good research, and a bad proposal well . . . not only gets you a bad grade, it also leads to bad research. You can show off your skills in paper writing and in referencing, and prove that you have critical thinking skills, through a good proposal.

What is a proposal for? (At BSc level, other levels may vary). It is to show:

- that you understand the basic elements of research
- that you can do a literature review
- that you understand ethics and ethical application in research
- that you understand how to think critically
- Oh . . . that you have an idea of something to look at that will make a difference to patient care.

A proposal answers the questions:

- What do you plan to get done?
- Why do you want to do it?
- How are you going to do it?
- What have others done, and how is yours different?

Answering those questions, you should show that your research idea is both unique and important, that you understand the relevant ideas, principles and literature, and that you understand and can apply a valid research methodology.

You will need more than research skills to pull off a good research proposal or paper – you also need writing skills. Be clear, concise and specific – write in academic voice, and try to keep your word count down. A good project might crash because of poor writing, poor spelling, poor grammar or incorrect format. Show your passion for the topic, but also be objective about the outcome.

The following box will help you with how it should be written, but, as explained above, the methodology stuff is up to you. In all of these points, remember how you look at research critically, and apply these questions to your own proposal. The same form is also downloadable from the Evolve website for this book (http://evolve.elsevier.com/siviter/studentnurse/).

Writing a research proposal

Title (10–15 words max)
- Be concise and descriptive. Don't say 'a study of' – just spit it out! If you are looking at the development of fingertip burns in smokers, say 'Fingertip burns in smokers: emergence of new plastic surgery techniques'
- Try to be informative but catchy – which would you rather read: 'Intimacy in the over 80s; benefits for cognition' or 'Sexy grannies keep grandpa thinking' (OK, that might be pushing it, but you get the idea!).

Abstract (300 words)
- Start with the research question, phrased as a statement
- Include the rationale, the hyptothesis, the method and main findings
- When discussing the method, include design, procedures, the sample and any instruments that will be used
- Mention pilots, permission, sample type and if there is anything striking in your literature review.

Introduction
- The main purpose of the introduction is to provide the necessary background or context for your research problem
- Put your research question forward in a clear and focused way
- Show your creativity and critical thinking
- Show the significance and importance of the topic
- Give a historical overview
- Give the contemporary, modern context – looking forward if applicable
- Who are the stake holders and key players, and where is the topic most often discussed (look at literature review)?
- In general, give a snapshot in full colour, showing the value and depth of your planned research.

Start with a general statement of the problem area, outline the specific research problem, and then justify why yet another study on this area is merited. Make sure you cover all of the following:
- State the purpose of the study
- Set the stage in such a way as to show its necessity and importance
- Give the rationale and show why it's worth doing this research
- Identify and outline major issues and key issues to be addressed
- Identify the specific thing you are looking at, and the variables you are considering
- State your theory (if you have one) or hypothesis (if you have one)
- Outline the boundaries of the research – what are you NOT looking at?
- Optionally, give the key concepts.

Writing a research proposal—cont'd

Literature review

The literature review can be part of the introduction section, but having it separate shows a thorough review. The literature review serves several important functions:

- It ensures that you are not 'reinventing the wheel'
- It gives credit to those who have influenced and informed you
- It shows your knowledge of the research problem
- It shows you understand the theoretical and research issues relevant to the question and your method
- It shows your ability to critically evaluate relevant information
- It shows you can integrate concepts and understand how things relate
- It gives insight into your approach to the topic
- It shows that what you are planning to do will fill gaps or clarify confusion.

Make sure your review:

- is organised and structured
- is focused and coherent
- is concise
- cites influential and key literature
- is up to date
- is critical
- avoids trivial references
- uses primary sources as much as possible
- uses the right kind of sources (you can only use the *Daily Mail* for so much . . .).

Organising your literature review:

- Use subheadings – identify key areas, themes, or topics, for example, area of research, method, sample choice, etc.
- Tell a story that is interesting.

Methods

How will you do this research?

- Prove your methodology is sound
- Prove you have considered ethics
- Give enough info that someone else could do this work without you
- Demonstrate that you understand alternative methods, but that your chosen method is best
- Explain why you are using qualitative or quantitative or mixed methods.

Continued

Writing a research proposal—cont'd

For quantitative studies, the method section typically consists of the following sections:

- Design – Is it a questionnaire study or a focus group? What kind of design have you chosen?
- Participants – Who will take part in your study? What kind of sampling procedure is used?
- Instruments – What kind of measuring instruments do you use? Why? Are they valid and reliable?
- Procedure – How will you carry out your study? What activities are involved? How long will it take?

Results

Obviously you do not have results at the proposal stage; however, you need to show that you have some idea of the kind of data you will get, what they might show, and how you will present the information so others can make good use of it.

Discussion

- Convince the reader that the research is important and should go forward
- Show that you have considered ethics, transparency and confidentiality
- communicate a sense of enthusiasm and confidence
- mention the limitations and weaknesses.

Common mistakes in proposal writing:

1. Didn't do references properly!
2. Didn't write the paper well
3. Didn't follow the guidance for content
4. Didn't frame the research question
5. Didn't outline the boundaries
6. Didn't show awareness of key issues
7. Didn't keep up to date
8. Didn't cite the most important studies
9. Didn't present the theoretical contributions of other papers
10. Didn't stay focused on the research question
11. Didn't stay concise – went into too much detail in the wrong places
12. Didn't put forth a good argument
13. Didn't keep apples with apples and oranges with oranges
14. Used too many or too few words

Reflective Practice and Portfolios

> *I am so reflective now, I glow in the dark!*
> *Post-registration nursing student*

In this chapter

- What is reflection?
- Reflective models
- Why reflection is important to practice
- Portfolios
- References

WHAT IS REFLECTION?

Reflection is the process through which you look at yourself and your practice objectively. It is the way you integrate theory and practice, and the way you grow and mature as a professional and as a person. It's how you transform yourself from a student into a nurse, and later how you transform yourself into an expert and competent practitioner. It's also how you prove that evolution to others like tutors, mentors and the NMC.

Reflection is not a process that you do just once – from now on it needs to become an active and ongoing part of your life as a nurse. It can be done on paper and, as such, can be used as proof for assignments. It should also be something you do in your head.

I want you to imagine something . . .

You are going out to a very important dinner. As you look in the mirror, you notice that your hair is messy and there is a giant stain on the front of your top. Do you:

- *Shave your head, rip off your clothes, wear a hessian sack and a rope around your waist, and hide from the world by moving into a cave on a deserted island off the coast of Sicily so no one will ever know about what a mess you have been?*

- *Go out looking a mess and lie to all your friends that the stain just got there and that your hair is a new trendy style?*

- *Go out looking the way you are without caring how you look?*
- *Fix the hair, change the top, check the mirror again and go out with confidence that you now look your best?*

I hope you would just fix what you saw was wrong and get on with a great night! That's what reflection is all about. Looking at yourself honestly and objectively, seeing what is wrong, fixing it and carrying on. It's an ongoing process.

You don't just look in the mirror once a day – you check how you look when you have a chance, and you look in the mirror when:

- you try on new clothes
- you get your hair cut
- you have eaten – to make sure that those little green bits don't stay stuck in your teeth
- you are facing something (or someone!) important that you want to look your best for
- something happens that you know has messed up your appearance, to see how bad it is.

It's the same with reflection. You reflect on your practice and on your skills when:

- you learn something new
- something has changed – a new placement area, new mentor, new module
- you have done something and you want to make certain you did everything the right way and for the right reasons
- you want to prove you are competent, have learned, or have gained skills, knowledge or experience
- you make a mistake, want to learn from it and prevent a similar mistake from happening again.

Reflection is *not* about:

- blaming anyone – yourself or anyone else
- berating yourself
- being overly critical
- complaining
- being superficial and holding back what you are really thinking and feeling.

Reflection *is* about:

- gaining confidence in what you do well
- recognizing when you could have done better

○ learning from your mistakes
○ learning about yourself and your behaviour
○ trying to see yourself as others see you
○ being self-aware
○ changing the future by learning from the past.

You are going to make mistakes. You are going to think those mistakes are irreparable. You're going to convince yourself that your only option is a career in the exciting world of fast food. But, with reflection, you can overcome problems and mistakes, and become a self-aware and competent nurse.

REFLECTIVE MODELS

Now that you know how important reflection is to your growth as a professional nurse, you have to learn how to do it. There are numerous models, but the place to start is with Gibbs.

Gibbs' (1988) Model of Reflection

1. Describe the activity or experience in objective detail.
2. Discuss and explore any feelings you were having at the time of the experience.
3. Evaluate the experience: what really happened? What was good about it? What was bad? What factors contributed to this event?
4. Analyse the experience: what can you learn from it?
5. Conclusion: what could you have done differently? Anything you wish you had done? Wish you hadn't done?
6. Action plan: what can you plan on doing in the future?

John's (1994) Model of Reflection

1. **Description:** write an objective account of what happened (as in Gibbs). Think 'What are the significant issues I need to pay attention to?' Then go through the experience, using different cues. Each cue should help you to tease the experience apart.
2. **Aesthetics** (the creative, interactive parts of the situation): ask yourself, 'Why did I act as I did? How did my actions affect other people (the patient, my colleagues, other people, myself)? How did other people feel about this situation? How do I know how they feel?'
3. **Personal** (your own thoughts and experiences): 'How was I feeling? What factors influenced me? What was going on in my head?'
4. **Ethics** (the rights and wrongs): 'Did I behave the way I think I should behave? Did I do anything out of character? Anything that makes me

feel guilty? Was there anything that made me behave differently than I usually would?'

5. **Empirical** (knowledge and information): 'What information and knowledge did I have or should I have had about this situation?'

6. **Reflexivity** (making sense of things; looking at the past to change the future): 'Does this situation remind me of past situations? What can I do differently in the future? If I did something differently, how would it be different for my patient, my colleagues, others or myself? How do I feel now about this situation? Can I support others better because of this situation and what I have learned? Has this changed the way I behave?'

It doesn't matter which model you use. I have given you the two basic ones here, but there are many more basic and advanced ones. You will probably adapt these models to a method that works best for you. It would be a really good idea to read about reflection in more detail. Some books are listed in the Useful Books, Journals and Other Resources section at the end of this book, in addition to the sources in the References section at the end of the chapter.

WHY REFLECTION IS IMPORTANT TO PRACTICE

The key to reflection working for you Is that you must be *absolutely* honest with yourself. You also have to eliminate the intense desire to involve (blame) other people. 'My mentor ignored me so I went off sick' isn't very useful. 'I was feeling afraid that I wouldn't pass the assessment, and I felt intimidated by my mentor, and I got myself worked up into believing that it would be OK to call in sick because I wanted to avoid having to cope with her' is much better. No one *makes* you do anything: you have to accept responsibility for the choices you make. Focus on *your* thoughts, feelings and reactions. Let other people worry about themselves. You can't change them, so don't waste your time trying: just learn from your experiences with them.

You can reflect on anything:

- Problems, mistakes and uncomfortable things
- Successes and achievements
- Journal articles
- Classroom sessions
- Conversations
- Television programmes
- Relationships
- Placement areas
- How to deal with a particular patient or colleague.

The point is: reflect on experiences that will either help you to grow or demonstrate that you have grown. Another idea is to look back through your reflections to when you were struggling, and reflect on things that show you have learned from past reflections.

So, it's time to get yourself a notebook and reflect. If you have a particularly good example of how you have changed or what you have learned, put it into your portfolio. It is a good idea to use your notebook as a reflective journal. Develop a pattern for yourself:

- Have a regular time and place to sit and reflect
- Keep the journal privately, so you can feel free to say whatever you need to without worrying about anyone else
- When you want to share a reflection, copy it from your journal
- Look back on past reflections periodically, and then reflect on how you are growing and maturing as a person and as a nurse
- Get used to reflecting on things in your head as well as on paper
- Write a reflection when you need to, as well as at your 'usual' time.

Reflection isn't the easiest thing you will do as a student, because it requires you to face some things that we all find a bit uncomfortable. Things like: 'I rushed because I wanted to leave early', or 'I was impatient because I had other things on my mind'. It's OK. We all have times when we do things for the wrong reasons; it's part of being human – and you are allowed to be human, even as a nurse.

Being a good nurse isn't as much about the mistakes you make (because you will make them, trust me!) as about how you learn from and handle those mistakes.

PORTFOLIOS

There are two different kinds of portfolio you might be concerned with as a nurse:

1. Student portfolios, both before and after registration. These show evidence of the academic and clinical achievements you need to complete a certain course.
2. Your PREP (post-registration education and practice) portfolio, which shows that you have met the criteria for ongoing registration.

Student portfolios

As a pre-registration student, your student portfolio is there for two main reasons:

1. For you and the university to keep track of your achievements
2. To see what you still need to get finished.

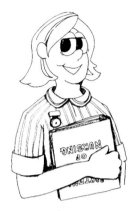

I didn't feel very confident until I looked back over my portfolio – then I saw how much I had accomplished. I didn't realize how far I had come – I'm getting good at being a nurse!

Third-year student nurse

A side-effect of your student portfolio is that it tells you what is important to you as a nurse. Notice how there is probably an area that talks about your ability to follow aseptic (sterile) technique, but nothing about how you make tea.

Pre-registration, it will seem like everyone in the world needs to look at your portfolio – mentors, personal tutors, even your friends. After you qualify, your portfolio is your own and you don't need to share it with anyone but the NMC. No-one but the NMC can force you to share the content of your portfolio with anyone else.

Your university will supply your student portfolio. It will contain lists of skills (or competencies) that you could develop and practise while on placement. It is up to *you* to know your portfolio, what is included in it, and what needs to be done during a specific placement. It is *not* up to your mentor or personal tutor to walk you through the portfolio reminding you of your obligations. It's *your* portfolio: you are in charge of whether or not it gets done.

Look through your portfolio before you go on a placement and try to identify areas that the placement could fulfil. (This is yet another reason to do a pre-placement visit and read up about the area in advance!) Plan how to get your needs met, and flag up areas you believe you might not achieve during the placement. Share this plan with your mentor, and ask for advice and support.

If you are concerned that you are not getting the opportunities you need, speak to your personal tutor and ask for help making your plan.

Keep a photocopy of essential things in your portfolio just in case something happens to it. If you pass a placement, photocopy the part where the mentor says you have passed. If anything ever happens to your portfolio, you still have proof.

Finally, don't see your portfolio as a burden. It's like a baby album – there are portraits of you as a baby nurse, all the way through your development into taking those first steps as a nurse. And, when you are a nurse, your days of keeping a portfolio have only just begun.

PREP (post-registration education and practice)

Your PREP portfolio is there:

1.   for you to keep track of achievements and learning
2.   to prove to the NMC that you are a competent practitioner who has kept up with the requirements for registration.

It's a while before you need to produce a PREP portfolio, but you can start to build one when you are a student. You can get a very useful publication called *The PREP Handbook* from the NMC.

You have an obligation to keep yourself up to date in nursing after you qualify, and your PREP portfolio is the way you do it. If you start your portfolio as a student, it can be very useful when you apply for a nursing job. So, this is what to do:

- Get yourself an A4 binder.
- Type up your CV as it stood before your nursing course.
- As you get attendance certificates for in-services or trainings, put them into the binder.
- For each assignment you do, write a brief synopsis and record your grade. If you fail, write up another one for the assignment that you submitted that passed and put a reflection about what you did differently!
- Write a brief synopsis about what you have learned in each module you take.
- Write a brief synopsis and reflection about every placement area you have.

Now, when you go to apply for a job, you have a lot of information about how you have prepared yourself to be a nurse. It's not a PREP folder really, because it's pre-registration, but it is the foundation for your eventual PREP. It gets you into the habit of saving things and being on the lookout for proof of your development.

Some of the nurses I know have done their PREP in interesting ways:

- One nurse started going to a gym for her own health, and kept a journal about her feelings so she could work out how to motivate her patients to increase their exercise. She reflected on how learning about exercise and how difficult it is to lose weight gave her more empathy with reluctant patients.
- Another nurse decided to stop smoking and kept a journal reflecting on what was difficult, how she felt and what was motivating her. She reflected on the process and outlined some ways she could help her patients to stop smoking.

- One elder care nurse did a weekly bank shift in A&E to keep her skills sharp. She reflected on the experiences she had there.
- One nurse reflected on the way nurses behaved on the TV programme *Holby City* and outlined issues with the *Code of Professional Conduct*!

You don't need to work desperately hard to keep up to date. It can be interesting and fun – the key is that you have to keep it relevant. As you go through your daily routines, think about how different things you may see or do could influence the way you do your nursing.

As the time comes for you to complete your course, there will probably be a lecture on how to do your portfolio. The *Nursing Standard* and the *Nursing Times* have both had good articles about portfolio development. Don't wait until the end to start your PREP portfolio: if you start it now, it will be yet another one of those good habits in nursing that you develop.

One part of your portfolio should be a review of research articles you have read, and reflections on how you brought them into practice. They don't have to be heavy, scholarly articles, but you should regularly be reading up-to-date information that is there to guide your practice.

If you never read, never change, never grow, then soon you will not be a nurse because you will have forgotten all the important things that make you a nurse, and when that happens, not only will you be unhappy in your job, but you will be one of those nurses that you as a student found so unpleasant to be with. Isn't it worth keeping up to date?

Summary

- Reflection is a process through which you grow and develop as a person and as a nurse.
- Reflection can be about good and bad things, and shouldn't be about blame or shame.
- Using a reflective model can guide you through the process of reflection more easily.
- You have to be honest with yourself for reflection to be effective.
- Your portfolio is yours, and you are responsible for making sure it is completed.
- You should know the expectations in your portfolio and plan for them to be met through your clinical placements.
- Keep copies of important bits of your student portfolio.
- Start keeping a record of what you do now, to help you start your PREP portfolio and to get into the good habit of paying attention to PREP.

REFERENCES

Gibbs, G., 1988. Learning by Doing: A Guide to Teaching and Learning Methods. Oxford Further Education Unit, Oxford

Johns, C., 1994. Guided reflection. In: Palmer, A., Burns, S., Bulman, C. (Eds.), Reflective Practice in Nursing. Blackwell Science, Oxford, pp. 110–130

11

Legal Issues for Students

In this chapter

- Records and record-keeping
- Disability and the Disability Discrimination Act/Equality Act
- The Data Protection Act
- The Health and Safety at Work Act
- Duty of care
- Consent
- Accountability
- Fitness for practice
- Negligence
- Bullying
- The Mental Capacity Act

Nursing is a profession full of legal issues. Having an understanding of those issues as a student will help you develop awareness and good practice for your future career. This is probably going to be a dull chapter – sorry – but these are important issues, and I promise that if you wade through this you will find that a lot of it is important and valuable. As always, if you need or want more information, go to the library, ask your personal tutor, check with your mentor, ask at the student union or call your union.

There are many legal issues that you will have to bear in mind as a student and as a nurse, but the areas outlined in this chapter are key basics for you. They are things of which you must constantly be aware; they are also things you will be assessed on, so knowing about them will help your grades.

RECORDS AND RECORD-KEEPING

Imagine that you have been brought to court. You are standing in the witness box and an intimidating barrister bellows, 'Student nurse! What did you get for your birthday in 1999?'

Would you be able to remember? You might remember some things, but certainly not all – especially the smaller things. Now imagine that the barrister then asks, 'And how were they wrapped? Were there bows? In what order did you open them? What time was it when you opened each item . . . ?'

Would you have the slightest inkling how to answer these questions completely and accurately? Probably not. Even though your birthday comes only once a year and is probably a significant event for you, most people can't remember every detail.

How then would you be able to remember every detail of things you did for patients on an average working day? You have to write them down! Writing things down is the only proof you will have that you did something, recognized something, said something . . . if you don't write it down, it never happened.

There are some key points to remember when writing things in patient notes:

- **The notes must be made in a timely manner.** If something significant happens, write it down as soon as possible afterwards.
- **Don't use abbreviations** except when the abbreviation will be absolutely clear to other readers.
- **Don't use slang or jargon.**
- **Write with a black, non-erasable pen.**

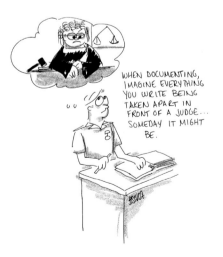

WHEN DOCUMENTING, IMAGINE EVERYTHING YOU WRITE BEING TAKEN APART IN FRONT OF A JUDGE... SOMEDAY IT MIGHT BE.

- **Never use Tippex™.** If you must correct an error, put a single line through it, write 'error' above it, initial it and carry on. If you write an entry in the incorrect patient's notes, cross through it, make another entry below it that says 'The above was entered incorrectly into the incorrect patient's notes', and sign it.

- **Have everything co-signed** by a qualified member of staff.

- **Be clear and specific.** Don't write 'Patient in pain; given meds'. Instead write, 'At 10 am patient complained of pain in the surgical area on a scale of 6/10. Given 10 mg of morphine orally at 10.20 am. At 11am patient said pain was much better and that no further medication was needed.' Write exactly what you did and when. You might be criticized for writing long notes but, legally, writing clear and specific notes is correct.

- **Be objective and non-judgemental.** Write your notes as if the person you are writing about is going to be reading them while sitting next to his or her solicitor. If you want to convey how someone is acting, simply repeat word for word what they tell you. Don't say someone is 'aggressive or violent'; instead say, 'Patient states "Get outta my face or I will kill you . . ."' If the patient swears, record the swear exactly. This tells others everything they need to know without you being accused of making a judgement. Don't say 'Patient was pouting'; instead say, 'Patient didn't make eye contact, appeared to be frowning, had arms crossed across chest, didn't answer when spoken to . . .' Describe what you see and what you hear, and let others reading it make up their own mind!

- **Don't leave blank areas** for other people to fill things in. Put a line through all empty space, then sign your name clearly.

- **Print your name clearly** if your signature is illegible. While you are a student, note 'student nurse' next to your name.

The following is a summary of good record-keeping, as outlined by the NMC.

Summary

Record-keeping is an integral part of nursing and midwifery practice:

- Good record-keeping is a mark of the skilled and safe practitioner.
- Records should not include abbreviations, jargon, meaningless phrases, irrelevant speculation or offensive subjective statements.
- Records should be written in terms that the patient or client can easily understand.
- By auditing your records, you can assess the standard of the record and identify areas for improvement and staff development.

- You must ensure that any entry you make in a record can easily be identified.
- Patients and clients have the right of access to records held about them.
- Each practitioner's contribution to records should be seen as of equal importance.
- You have a duty to protect the confidentiality of the patient and client record.
- Patients and clients should own their healthcare records as far as it is appropriate and as long as they are happy to do so.
- The principle of the confidentiality of information held about your patients and clients is just as important in computer-held records as in all other records.
- The use of records in research should be approved by your local Research Ethics Committee.
- You must use your professional judgement to decide what is relevant and what should be recorded.
- Records should be written clearly and in such a manner that the text cannot be erased.
- Records should be factual, consistent and accurate.
- You need to assume that any entries you make in a patient or client record will be scrutinized at some point.
- Good record-keeping helps to protect the welfare of patients and clients.

DISABILITY AND THE DISABILITY DISCRIMINATION ACT (NI) or EQUALITY ACT (GB)

What is a disability? A disability is a health condition or physical issue that makes things more difficult for someone. It can be something like sensory loss, learning disability, a disease like diabetes, or mobility problems. It can be temporary or permanent. It can affect the person visibly or invisibly. If people feel that there are things about their health that make it more difficult for them to do ordinary everyday things, then they are 'disabled', and are covered under disability legislation. That, however, doesn't mean they have ceased being *people*, worthy of respect and dignity, and capable of fruitful lives and careers!

In reality, disability isn't what happens as a result of an illness or problem – it's what happens when the rest of the world can't seem to cope with the way somebody needs to do things.

Don't feel 'badly' for disabled people – if you see someone who you think is disabled, don't pity them, and don't just help them without asking. It's nice to ask – but if you just assume they can't do something you are not giving them fair credit and you are likely to cause offence.

The key to legislation – about bullying, about disability, about consent – is all about the same thing: allowing people to have the right to make decisions, to have access to the same things as everyone else, and to enjoy their life in the way they want to.

The Acts give guidance about disabled people and set out their rights. For example, people who are disabled have a right to reasonable accommodation. That means that they have a right to work, and that their employers have to help them, supporting them by making reasonable changes (ones that aren't so big and expensive that it would put them out of business) to allow them to work.

There are disabled parking spaces, ramped floors and kerbs, wider doorways, and push buttons to open doors. There are also special considerations when applying for jobs, and extra support, like that available through Jobcentre Plus's 'Access to Work' programme. These are all because disabled people have the right to do whatever anyone else does – shop, work, go out to eat, progress in their chosen career, buy nice things – and it's not right to prevent them just because they can't physically get to the place, or because their 'vision' is provided by a guide dog, or because they speak British Sign Language instead of English. Disabled people cope – if an able-bodied person can't cope, who is really disabled? Here's a twist for you – did you realize that deaf people have their own language, their own culture, and some of them look at 'us' as disabled because we have to rely on hearing and can't enjoy the depth and complexity of *their* culture? What do you think about that?

The thing you need to remember is that disability is in the environment; it's the obstacle or the perception that prevents independence– it's not the *person*. Don't label people as disabled: the obstacles they face are not *who* they are as *people*.

And, as an aside to my comment about deaf culture above– this may not apply to everyone with hearing impairment, as even groups of people within larger groups show diversity. The best thing is to never judge a person; just to see each as a wonderfully unique and original individual, physically, spiritually, emotionally, culturally. It's all we each want to be, isn't it?

The absence of disabled parking is a good example of disability being exacerbated by lack of consideration on the part of the able-bodied. Having accessible parking makes going out less of an obstacle because it allows the disabled person to park close and open the doors enough to get out of the car along with whatever equipment is needed. But, if once you get to the shop you can't get in, where does that leave you? There was a disabled lady who sued a store because their sale items were on the first floor and there was no lift – she alleged that she was discriminated against because she couldn't shop there. Disability legislation is there to help remove the obstacles that are unfairly and unreasonably put into place because people don't understand that disabled people are capable, competent and strong, or...weak, incompetent and confused...just like everyone else.

The lesson is, don't add disability to a disabled person's life by your attitude, your lack of understanding, or even your well-meaning but ill-advised desire to help. Would I refuse the offer of a door held open for me? No. Would I ask for help if needed? Yes. Be available, be willing, but let people do for themselves what they can, and treat them as you would anyone else – with dignity, respect and compassion.

Let me share something that means a lot to me . . . 'Dee' is a patient who is a nurse and who has suffered a brain injury. She has no movement or sensation down her left side following a stroke during a routine operation. When she was admitted, she was angry and pushed staff away, bitter (quite reasonably!) because, as a nurse, she felt guilty accepting care no matter how badly she needed it. Because I too face challenges, we were on an even field – she wasn't bitter about me walking, because I wasn't: she could trust me. She knew I knew – we had an instant rapport. She was angry, she was hurt, and I could help because I could relate to her feelings. That's what I mean about my 'disability' giving me things – I had credibility, because I have the tee-shirt – or, uhm the crutches – to prove that I have been where my patient is going. If having a spinal-cord injury makes me a better nurse, then it's not really a disability, is it?

The Acts are about access, but also about how people are treated. It is not right to behave towards anyone in a way that makes him or her feel harassed, bullied or treated unfairly just because of a disability. It's about attitude – people can behave in very demeaning or belittling ways, sometimes without even knowing – like the person who always greets the guide dog rather than the person at the other end of the leash. I have even been patted, much like one pats a good child on the head as a reward . . . it not only makes me feel like I am an inch tall, it also makes my pain level go through the roof because my back is very tender to touch. Does the person patting me or the person addressing the dog instead of the blind person (yes, I said blind, not vision impaired, not retinally challenged, but blind – quick, hide under the table, the sky is about to fall!) mean to belittle anyone? Probably not – but in the law, it's how the disabled person feels that matters, not what you *meant*.

The Acts make this type of treatment illegal, a violation of the person's human rights. So, next time you eye that tasty space next to the shop's front door, leave it for the person who needs it more than you want it. Try to remember to say 'can I help you or are you OK?' before assuming a disabled person needs help . . . and, if you are really nervous or intimidated, try saying 'could you talk to me about why you need to use that scooter? I don't mean to be nosy, but I would like to understand more . . . ' instead of making a comment. Respect goes a long way.

As a nurse, though, there are some other special considerations of the Acts: you have to make sure that people are not disadvantaged in their care because of their disability. Remember your role as a patient advocate? This is where it really comes into play: if you hear someone making fun of your patient because of his or her disability, it's up to you to speak up; if you notice that some people can't make use of services because of their disability, then again speak up. There was a counselling centre at one of the local hospitals, but it had no disabled parking. When asked why not, they said it was because it was a staff-only counselling centre and there were no disabled staff. What could you do in that case?

Every employer is mandated to have a disability rights officer – someone obligated to make sure that the disability legislation is met, and that people's human rights are protected. Although that protection may start with you as a nurse, it is the obligation of your entire organization to protect the disabled. Remember – disability is really when someone else puts an obstacle in place that doesn't need to be there, or when someone leaves an obstacle in a place where it shouldn't be . . . it is less about the reason the obstacle is a problem than it is about the willingness of the rest of the world to be considerate.

For more about disability issues, check out the BBC's *Ouch!* pages: they are resources for disability issues, with frequently asked questions and many good links.

THE DATA PROTECTION ACT

The Data Protection Act (1998) basically boils down to two simple principles:

1. You cannot share any information about someone without his or her permission.
2. Any information you get from someone has to be used in accordance with the reason he or she gave it to you to begin with.

If, while you are a student, you leave your telephone number with the ward for staff to call you if there are any problems, and they use it to call you when your placement has finished to see if you would like to work a shift, this would be seen as a violation of the Data Protection Act unless you told someone it was OK for them to call you for shifts. If they were to give your phone number to another ward, and you didn't know about it and didn't consent, that would also be a violation. Giving your telephone number to a patient's family is certainly a violation!

Basically, people who hold data (called 'data controllers' in the Act) have an obligation to keep the data in accordance with the law and only use them within the correct context.

As a student, you need to be aware that giving out personal information about a patient (or a colleague) could be a problem:

- **Always check with the patient:** 'Mandy, there is a Jane Gardiner on the phone, she says she is your friend and wants to know how you are. What should I tell her?' Perhaps you can't ask the patient; if the person calling is a real friend or family member, he or she will understand if you need to explain that you can't give out any information. Offer to take a message and pass it on to the patient. If the patient is critically ill, or in serious condition, pass the call to a more senior nurse.

- **Don't ever give out *any* staff information:** 'I'm sorry, I cannot give you any information about the off-duty or who is working on the ward. You may speak to the ward manager – would you like me to see if she is available?'

- **If you aren't sure what information it is OK to divulge, ask someone.**

You might keep notes from handover, and perhaps even information about patients you have cared for, in your pocket. Don't; it could be used against you. What if someone else, someone who doesn't have the right to that information, finds your scraps of paper? Always destroy, and don't take home, any information about patients. How would Shelly Croghan feel if she knew her nurse had dropped something in the market and someone read it – only to find out that 'Give Shelley Croghan a suppos because she's constipated' was the order of the day? Trust – it's all about being worthy of trust.

In the course of working with people, and because you are a student collecting data, you will come across opportunities where the interaction could serve as evidence for your portfolio. You have no automatic right. As we discussed in patient confidentiality, if you need information about a patient for an assignment or your portfolio, you have to make absolutely sure that:

- no-one could identify the patient, or the trust, ward or hospital, from your materials
- you have the patient's consent to use the information.

Not taking care of these two considerations could get you into trouble.

If you feel that, during a placement, your rights under the Data Protection Act have been abused, then you should go to the university, the student union or your union for help.

THE HEALTH AND SAFETY AT WORK ACT

The Health and Safety at Work Act (1974) is a complex one, but there are three basic principles:

1. **Employers** have an obligation to provide a working environment that does not pose a health or safety risk to employees, and, if there are any

risks that are present because of the nature of the work, protective equipment must be supplied by the employer to protect the employee from risk.

2. **Employees** have an obligation to avoid risk, to be aware of and act in accordance with health and safety protocols and policies, and to notify the appropriate representative of the employer if they become aware of a risk or hazard. If an employee does something that is a violation of the policies, he or she is liable for whatever happens.

3. **Employers and employees** have an obligation to protect non-employees from risk.

What does this mean for you as a nursing student? It means that:

- you have an obligation to know and follow all relevant health and safety policies, including manual handling, and as an agent of the employer you have an obligation to be aware of how hazards in the environment could affect other people
- if you choose to ignore a policy and either yourself or someone else is harmed, you are in trouble
- if you see a hazard and don't tell anyone about it, you could be in trouble, especially if someone else gets hurt
- you have a right to have the appropriate protective equipment – aprons, gloves that fit, etc.

Health and safety is a huge issue in the NHS. There are mandatory trainings and policies to follow. Here is how to be certain you are following them:

- **Stay awake and pay attention** during your mandatory health and safety lectures!
- **Know how to be safe.** On your first day in a placement area, or on your pre-placement visit if possible, make yourself familiar with fire exits, location of fire extinguishers, how to call for help in an emergency, and where any emergency call buttons are. *You must have this information before you do anything else on that ward.*
- **Find out the location of the health and safety policies.**
- **Know what you are doing.** If there is any equipment with which you are not familiar, don't use it until you have been properly taught.
- **Protect yourself.** If you need different size gloves, latex-free gloves, or any other personal protection equipment, let someone know and don't work until you have what you need.
- **Be sharp-smart.** Be aware of the location of sharps boxes and follow sharps disposal policy. Don't *ever* walk around with a sharp in your hand. Don't *ever* recap a syringe. Take a sharps box with you when you do an injection or use a needle. If you get stuck or stabbed, you *must* report it – your health and career are on the line.

- **Know the environment.** On your pre-placement visit, ask if there are any special health and safety risks in that placement area, and, if there are, what procedures are in place for protection. Is there special equipment you will need or need to use? Are there special policies and procedures that will need to be followed? Do any patients require any kind of special care?

- **Be aware of biohazard materials.** Handle and dispose of biohazard materials in the appropriate way. If you have any doubts, ask someone to help you. Don't put sharp or potentially sharp (e.g. glass tubes, bottles, IV bags with plastic spikes) items in plastic bin bags. Wash your hands!

- **Wash your hands!!!** I know I've said this already, but it is crucial in health and safety.

- **Follow manual-handling policy.** If you hurt your back as a student, that's it. Your career is over, you have no recourse to any work injury benefits, and you will never be physically the same.

- **Just say no.** If you find yourself put into a situation where you don't feel you can be safe, remove yourself. This includes 'specialing' patients (i.e. supervising one-to-one), lifting, or using equipment you don't know how to use. It also applies when you don't have the protective equipment you need. You have a right to say 'I can't do that'.

It all boils down to protecting yourself, your patients and your colleagues, being aware of risks and of how to protect yourself, and following the policies in place for your protection. Don't ever go beyond the limitations of your role as a student.

DUTY OF CARE

To the average person, someone dressed in a uniform so that she looks like a nurse *is* a nurse. That person will expect a certain standard from you, and will expect that, as a nurse, you have the knowledge and skills to help. If you are on your way to or from a placement in your uniform, you need to be aware that you could be identified as a nurse (most people won't see a difference between a nurse and a student nurse) and expected to help a person in distress. If you let friends, family and neighbours know you are a nursing student, then they might also expect you to help if they get into trouble. You need to make it clear that you are a student, not a nurse. You might be very experienced, but you have to accept the limitations of your role as a student. You must make sure that you never act as a nurse without supervision by a qualified nurse. You must make absolutely certain that people know you are a nursing student and that being a student is not the same as being a nurse.

Duty of care means living up to the standards and expectations held for you, by the NMC and by the general public, as a nurse. It means that you:

- can't just go home when your job is done if there is no one to take over your workload
- can't go to lunch or on break if there is no one to cover
- are a nurse 24 hours a day.

Duty of care also means that you have an obligation to uphold the NMC code of professional conduct and *not* to act in a way that could bring discredit to nursing as a profession.

As a student, your duty is less because you are not a nurse, but you must remember that patients, their families, and sometimes other professionals, will not necessarily realize that you are a student. It is your responsibility to not take on tasks beyond the scope of your role as a student.

CONSENT

There are two kinds of consent:

1. Implied consent
2. Expressed consent.

Implied consent

Implied consent means you assume that, based on circumstances and the situation, a person would want you to help. If someone is unconscious, for example, you don't need to wait until he or she gives you permission to start doing cardiopulmonary resuscitation (CPR)! Implied consent also means that some things are expected of you in your role. Patients expect that you will know how to move and handle them properly; you don't need to get a signed consent form every time you boost them up the bed. If you are in a situation where you know that, although unable to give expressed consent, a patient has not already indicated that he or she *doesn't* want a particular action taken on his or her behalf, and you believe that a reasonable person would want a certain action taken, then that is implied consent.

Expressed consent

Expressed consent is when a patient actively says 'I want this', knowing the possible complications, side-effects and consequences of the decision. Usually this means signing a form, but in some emergency situations a doctor or other professional can take consent verbally and ask for those present to witness the consent. Patients' consent should always be *informed consent*.

Informed consent

This means that someone has explained to patients in clear, non-medical language what is happening to them, and for what the consent is being sought. It means that patients make decisions about what happens to them with all the information necessary to really understand the impact that decision will have on their life and health. This means that people who are not able to make competent decisions really can't give consent.

Adults who suffer from an illness or disability that impairs their ability to take in or understand information can have a legal guardian appointed to make decisions for them. You can't assume that family members have a right to make decisions on another person's behalf, even husband and wife. There is no automatic legal right for next of kin to make a decision about a loved one.

Adults with a temporary inability to understand the consequences of a decision or refusal to accept care have to be dealt with carefully. In some cases, their refusal to receive care will be over-ridden after their inability to make a competent decision is well documented. At other times there will be legal involvement. As a student you should never allow yourself to get into a situation involving issues of consent, because they can get very contentious and you really aren't in a position to do anything to help anyway. You should find a qualified nurse who has the accountability and experience to make certain that the patient's rights and health are both protected.

Another issue that involves consent is making sure that a patient really has given informed consent. Before you participate in any procedure for which the patient has given consent, make sure that the patient really does know what is happening. As a student this isn't as much of an issue, but if you have any reason to suspect that the patient doesn't understand what is happening and thus really hasn't given consent, then you have an obligation to bring that concern immediately to a staff nurse, your mentor, a sister or another nurse.

The other side of consent is that patients have the right to say 'No'. Just as you have to make sure you have the patient's consent to do something, you must respect a patient who says 'No'. But, just as consent must be informed consent, any refusal must also be an informed refusal. You have an obligation as a nurse to make absolutely certain that the patient knows the consequences of the decision to refuse care. You also must be able to tell the difference between someone saying 'I don't want that . . . ' because he or she needs reassurance, and someone saying 'You will not do that to me' because he or she really will not allow you to do something. If as a student you are worried that a patient is refusing treatment, step back and don't proceed. Get help and support from your mentor or another nurse. It's something you will deal with more effectively as you gain experience.

ACCOUNTABILITY

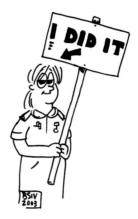

Accountability means that you are willing to stand up and say, 'Yes I did that'. Professional accountability means that you are willing for your practice to be examined closely and that you are willing to be honest about what you do and why. It means that you as a nurse can say that you uphold the highest standards of professional nursing care.

As a student, you are not yet 'accountable'. A qualified nurse is accountable under the Code of Conduct, but you are merely 'responsible' for your behaviour. You must behave in a way that demonstrates that you are thoughtful and responsible, but a qualified nurse must act to a higher standard. You are not yet expected to uphold the highest standards of professional nursing care because you are still a student, and students will make more mistakes than others. That's why you are a student!

An essential aspect of qualified nurses' accountability is that when you, as a student, work with them, they are accountable for what you may do. That's why they supervise you; because what you do will reflect on them. If you do something under supervision that turns out to be wrong (like making a medication error) then the nurse – not you – is the one in trouble as long as you behaved responsibly and within the limits of your education and role as a student. Their training, education and experience give them a greater level of responsibility.

FITNESS FOR PRACTICE

As a student and as a nurse you have an obligation to be fit for practice. Quite simply, you cannot work as a nurse if you are not emotionally, psychologically or physically fit to do so. Some people are physically injured; others suffer from stress or an illness that interferes with their ability to nurse. Some nurses change to a different type of nursing (for example, working for NHS Direct) when illness or injury makes it too difficult for them to work with patients in the clinical area.

You know how you shouldn't drive when you are drunk? Or how you will have to hand back your driving licence if you lose your sight? Well, it's the same in nursing. If you are ever too stressed, too ill or too injured to work, it is your obligation to let someone know. You must tell your university and you can make an appointment to see someone in the occupational health department.

You must never attend a placement or work a shift when you have been drinking or if you are using recreational drugs. Even some drugs prescribed by your GP could interfere with your judgement. You must be certain that nothing impairs your ability to make the best decisions possible for your patients. Just as you shouldn't drive a car if you are impaired, so you cannot nurse people when you are not able to give your best to care for them. There is no sin in needing to take time to take care of yourself. You can't be the nurse your patients need you to be if you are on the verge of being a patient yourself!

Part of fitness for practice is more than being physically and emotionally well; it's also about being of good character. Can you be a therapeutic nurse who mugs people in her spare time? No. Because, as a nurse, you have access to privileged information and intimate details about people's lives, and because people trust you, you must be a person who is above question. To be fit for practice you must be of sufficiently good character to uphold the trust placed in you.

So, if you get into trouble during your course – are arrested or commit a serious traffic offence – talk to someone at your union or student union and let them know so they can help you make sure it doesn't prevent you from becoming a nurse. Some offences will make it impossible for you to qualify, but most things that cause students' problems are silly things that got out of control.

NEGLIGENCE

Negligence is a legal term that means someone didn't do something that he or she should have done and now that person is liable for the damage the action (or inaction) caused. To be proved negligent, four things must be true:

1. There must be a duty of care present
2. There must be a breach of that duty (either an act of commission or an act of omission)
3. It must be foreseeable that a breach of duty could cause harm
4. Harm must result.

We've already talked about duty of care (the expectation that you will behave in a certain way and that you will not abandon a patient); a breach in duty of care means that you either do something wrong, or don't do something you should do. If you breach your duty of care, and you know that a breach could mean that the patient comes to harm, and the patient actually comes to harm, then you are negligent.

One test used when thinking about negligence is the Bolam test. This basically asks you to think about what most other practitioners just like you would do in a similar situation. If you are acting as most other reasonable practitioners would act in similar circumstances, then you meet the conditions of the Bolam test and are not negligent.

Negligence is scary, and that's why it's so important for you to understand what your duty of care is. As a student, it's unlikely you would ever be named as negligent because you are working under the direct supervision of a qualified nurse. But if you are ever worried that a potential act or omission could harm someone, you must let your mentor or another nurse know.

BULLYING

Bullying can be a serious issue for students and staff alike. There is no easy way to deal with bullies, but there is one thing that you should remember to help you through . . .

It's not your fault if a bully decides to pick on you. There is nothing you could have or should have done differently, it's not your fault and you are not to blame. You are not being bullied because you are weak, and you certainly don't deserve it.

There are some ways to handle being bullied:

- Recognize that if the bully were really as powerful and important as he or she is trying to make you believe, he or she wouldn't need to resort to bullying to get things done.
- Realize that bullies are really afraid of working with and coping with other people, and act the way they do because they feel inadequate as people.
- Reflect on what happens.
- Don't believe what bullies say. Don't let them into your head.
- Don't try to fix bullies. They are not your problem.

If you feel you are being bullied, go to someone for help immediately. Document what is happening, reflect and try to pinpoint the behaviour that makes you feel bullied. Often, simply standing up to the bully in a gentle way is enough:

I don't like being spoken to in that way.

Sometimes, you might even need to say:

It feels as though you are trying to bully me, and I am not going to tolerate it.

Sometimes, however, you won't be able to say anything at all. Sometimes the person might be your mentor, or another nurse, colleague, professional or even a patient.

Bullying will destroy your spirit if you allow it to continue. It can erode your confidence and stress you out. It is also wrong and illegal. So, if you find yourself being bullied, re-read what I said above about it not being your fault. Get help and support from friends, colleagues, at university, through the student union and through your union. If you see someone else being bullied, support that person and stand up for him or her.

I can't help any more than this in a couple of paragraphs, but what I will tell you is this:

- You don't have to suffer alone; it's important to talk about feeling bullied
- Bullying is wrong; it is *not* the victim's fault
- Bullies are people who can't cope with people in the normal, appropriate ways
- If you are the victim of a bully, there is nothing wrong with you except that you are someone who the bully envies, and bullies can't handle someone being good when they feel so bad about themselves.

Remember, document, reflect and go for help as soon as you recognize there is a problem. The Royal College of Nursing has published an excellent booklet for nursing students about bullying and harassment.

THE MENTAL CAPACITY ACT

Who the Mental Capacity Act affects

The Mental Capacity Act (2005) affects everyone aged 16 and over, and provides a legal framework to empower and protect people who may not be able to make some decisions for themselves – for example, people with a brain injury, mental health problems, dementia, learning disabilities, stroke or neurological problem.

Key parts of the Act are as follows:

- Everyone has the right to make decisions for him- or herself, and to determine the path his or her life should take.
- Because of problems, some people simply do not have the ability to make the decisions that are their right to make. This doesn't mean they have less of a right – only that they don't have the capacity to make decisions.
- Ultimately, it may be a court that has to make a decision for a person with diminished capacity.
- When it comes to capacity in a healthcare setting, it is important to consider the type of issue . . . is there a difference between getting consent so you can give a pain tablet, and getting consent for open-heart surgery? Yes, and that means that doctors and other healthcare professionals have

to be aware of the consequences and risks of some decisions, and handle consent and capacity in those areas more carefully.

- If a person can meet two tests, that person can make a decision for him- or herself: the person has (a) to understand the decision, including understanding fully the consequences involved, and (b) to be able to weigh information, using judgement and reason to come up with a decision.

- When, in the healthcare environment, a person is seen as perhaps not able to consent, an appropriate professional, often a doctor, has to determine if that person is able to consent. If he or she lacks capacity, it should be documented why the assessor believes this is the case.

- A doctor's assessment may be necessary before consent for a medical treatment or procedure, before a legal decision is made or a signature is witnessed, or before court proceedings about capacity, as insight into the persons' medical condition may explain the reason capacity is diminished.

- The doctor or individual assessing capacity has to think about whether the capacity is diminished permanently or temporarily – and if it is possible to wait for the time when the person can make a decision on his or her own behalf.

- Lack of capacity is not the same as lack of communication. Where a person needs support to communicate, perhaps through speech and language therapy, or even through a psychology professional, every attempt must be made to help that person communicate his or her decision. Not being able to tell someone what he or she wants isn't the same as not being able to decide.

- Medical care can be delivered in the absence of consent when it is medically necessary and seen as being in the patient's best interest, weighing the risks, benefits and outcomes.

- 'Best interest' is something that goes beyond health; it extends into spirituality, culture, emotions, dignity, quality of life, relationships and financial welfare. It's not about what is easier on the carers; it's genuinely what the person would likely choose for him- or herself if he or she were able – not what we want the person to choose for our benefit.

- No one – not even a parent (after majority), a spouse or a child – has the automatic right to give consent for anyone else, and no one should ever sign a consent form on behalf of another, unless there is a legal order in place that allows them to do so.

- There is a principle called the doctrine of necessity which states that if something is necessary to preserve life or prevent deterioration, then, unless there is evidence that the person would refuse, we should assume he or she would consent.

- Although everyone has a right to confidentiality, sometimes this has to be balanced with the necessity of finding out what someone would want. It may be necessary to give some information to family in order to ask if they have an opinion about what a person would choose, but the person disclosing information needs to be cautious and keep confidentiality in mind.

- In some cases, a person might choose to make an advance statement – sometimes called an advance directive – that sets out his or her wishes in case that person is not able to make his or her own decision.
- Although healthcare professionals are not legally bound to *provide* care requested by an advanced directive, they are legally bound to honour a *refusal* to give consent as long as the person making the advanced directive met the criteria for capacity when the advanced directive was prepared, and there is no evidence the person was coerced or forced into refusing, and they must honour the refusal even if they, or family members, disagree.
- When necessary, the High Court can determine consent on an individual's behalf.
- People who lack capacity to make decisions are especially vulnerable to exploitation or abuse, and healthcare professionals should be especially vigilant to protect vulnerable people.

The Mental Capacity Act is a complex act, but its goal is simple: people who can at any level determine the course of their own life should be able to do so, and individuals who cannot should have support in order to live as they would choose by there being robust arrangements in place to make sure that decisions are always made in accordance with what individuals would probably decide for themselves and along with what is holistically in their best interest.

In addition to searching for Mental Capacity Act in a search engine, organizations like Help the Aged, Age Concern, SCOPE, MENCAP, Motor Neuron Association, etc., all have information about mental capacity. You can read more about the MCA 2005 at the website for the National Archives: www.legislation.gov.uk/ukpga/2005/9/contents

Summary

- Record-keeping is an integral part of nursing and midwifery practice.
- Good record-keeping is a mark of the skilled and safe practitioner.
- Information should only be shared when the person giving the information is aware that it may be shared, and should only be shared if it's shared in accordance with the reason it was divulged – for example, if a person gives his or her information to get a doctor's appointment, it can't be used to try to sell that person windows.

- People have a right to enjoy the life they choose, and as nurses we have an obligation to support them (ACTS), support their right to consent or to have decisions made on their behalf, if they are not able to consent, that are in their best interest (MCA 2005).
- No one can consent on behalf of another person.
- No one has a right to information about anyone else.
- No one has a right to make anyone else feel inferior, belittled, harassed, unwanted or vulnerable.
- Nurses are obliged to maintain fitness for practice: failure to be fit for practice can cause someone to lose the right to be a nurse.
- Negligence is when a person with a duty of care fails to live up to that duty and, as a result, harm that could be anticipated actually occurs.
- Qualified nurses are accountable for their acts of omission and commission – what they do and what they fail to do – and this means that they have a duty of care. The Code of Conduct specifies that nurses must acknowledge their limitations – a nurse with limitations who fails to do something to fix those limitations is guilty of failure to live up to the code.
- Consent requires an understanding of the consequences and risks, as well as the ability to weigh facts to make a decision.
- Health and Safety is a shared obligation – the employee, employer and public must work sensibly together to make things work. Assessing risks, identifying hazards and putting things in place to avoid injury are all key.

REFERENCES

Data Protection Act, 1998. (Confidentiality and information.)
Dimond, B., 2004. Legal Aspects of Nursing, 4th ed. Longman, London.
Health and Safety in the Workplace, 1974.
Mental Capacity Act, 2005.
Mental Health Act, 2007. (Deals with consent quite intensively.)
Tingle, J., Cribb, A., 2007. Nursing Law and Ethics, 3rd ed. Wiley Blackwell, Oxford.

Websites

www.dca.gov.uk/legal-policy/mental-capacity/guidance.htm
www.nmc-uk.org

Final Thoughts

It seems so long ago that I wrote the first "final thoughts" . . . I thanked you for buying this book. I told you that I hoped it would encourage you, help you stay on your course and become a nurse – and I was overwhlemed with the responses and feedback we received. Thank you to all those who have bought this book – not only buying it, but for telling your friends about it, and for making it such a part of your preparation for becoming a nurse. You have treated me very well, and allowed me to share your successes and concerns.

You told the publisher that the book was a friend, a reliable resource to help you settle into your course, and that you found it encouraged and inspired you. I spoke to so many students who had purchased the book – either through email, or through professional events – and the stories were the same: students had been touched by the book, and this pleased me more than I can say.

I have tried to explain things as if you were my own student and I was your mentor. And even though I don't know you by name, I feel like I know who you are. You may not always feel it, but nurses do care about you – they just don't always show it because there are so many things going on, but we *are* glad to have you. And I would like to apologize for us all in advance for those times when you need us to show you we understand but we are too busy to notice. The men and women who have become nurses are a good group of people and we really are looking forward to you joining us. But, you have to survive your course first.

Don't give up on yourself. Be patient with friends and family who are struggling to get through your course almost as much as you are! Lean on your friends in the course and let them know they can lean on you. Say thank you to mentors and tutors who really make a difference so you can encourage them to keep working so hard. Don't let a bad grade or a bad experience knock your confidence. Don't hide it when you need help, and don't be silent when you should speak up for yourself. Don't allow abuse, harassment or bullying to ruin your spirit – get help when its needed.

Your success depends not on your academic ability, your experience in health care, or even on your overall 'nursiness'. Those who finish the course do it because they were the ones who didn't give up. That's why I want to give you these final thoughts:

'Nothing in the world can take the place of persistence. Talent will not; nothing is more common than unsuccessful men with talent. Genius will not; unrewarded genius is almost a proverb. Education will not; the world is full of educated derelicts. Persistence and determination are omnipotent. The slogan 'press on' has solved and will solve the problems of the human race.'

(Calvin Coolidge, 30th President of the United States of America)

The NHS is changing. It needs you more than ever—to be patient, compassionate and kind. It needs you to persevere, to show real stamina, insight and willingness to be something special. It needs good nurses.

And that's where I leave you – press on. Some days you will want to hide and cry, others you will just wish you could stay in bed. You will have sleepless nights and stress-filled weekends. But I promise that the good will outweigh the bad and you will be through the course before you know it. Just keep putting one foot in front of the other. Press on!

Bethann

Useful Books, Journals and Other Resources

SUGGESTED BOOKS AND RESOURCES

I have read or used each of these books, either in the current or an older edition. I have hundreds of nursing books; I have recommended those I believe will help you the most. But before you buy a book, look at it in the library and try to decide if the value the book will give you is worth the cover price. Some are worth buying; others are more useful if you just borrow them occasionally.

I believe that most of the books I have listed here are worth buying (feel free to copy this and send it out as a Christmas or birthday list) because you will get your money out of them as a student and some you will be able to use as a nurse as well.

I prefer to buy my books new, so I can take care of them and keep them in good condition, but you can buy books second-hand, sometimes at your university, but also from eBay (www.ebay.com) and Amazon (www.amazon.co.uk). Be aware that second-hand books might not be the most current edition and might not be in great condition.

A note about websites – they go out of date very quickly, so I haven't put many here. There are hundreds of useful sites; when you find a good one, share it with your colleagues.

Finally, I haven't referred to books that are specific to the four branches. You will have time during your common foundation programme to find out which books are most useful – through your lecturers, library, and students who are ahead of you in the branch.

Bullying

www.bullying.co.uk
This website is mainly directed at school children, but also contains information that is relevant to adults.

Clinical skills

Jamieson, E., McCall, J., Whyte, E., 2007. Clinical Nursing Practices. Churchill Livingstone, Edinburgh
A good basic book that explains the procedures every nurse needs to know, from basics like how to take a temperature, to more complicated procedures like how to assist at a liver biopsy. It reflects on the activities of living categories for each procedure. It is a 'must' for a new student who is inexperienced in healthcare, and is also useful for more experienced students who are transitioning from an HCA to a nursing role.

Skinner, S., 1998. Understanding Drug Therapies. Baillière Tindall, London
A good book to help you understand different drug classes and how they act. Easy to read but thorough.

Walsh, M., Ford, P., 1989. Nursing Rituals, Research and Rational Actions. Heinemann, Oxford
An old book that you can get second-hand from eBay or Amazon. I found it very enlightening and useful. It discusses the reasons we do things as nurses, and is written in a personable and enjoyable way.

Mallett, J., Dougherty, L., 2004. The Royal Marsden Hospital Manual of Clinical Nursing Procedures, sixth edn. John Wiley & Sons, Oxford
Also simply called 'The Marsden Manual', this gives step-by-step outlines, including rationales and explanations, for most nursing procedures. It is a definitive guide to clinical practice and, although not cheap, is a good investment.

Common foundation programme

Kenworthy, N., Snowley, G., Gilling, C., (eds) 2002. Common Foundation Studies in Nursing, third edn. Churchill Livingstone, Edinburgh
Great book, offers in-depth information about essential topics. It will guide you through your common foundation programme.

Brooker, C., Waugh, A., (eds), 2007. Foundations of Nursing Practice. Fundamentals of Holistic Care. Mosby, Edinburgh
This book is specifically for the common foundation programme, but you will use it throughout your course. It covers all branches of nursing, and includes material that is both common to all and specific to each branch. All the basic concepts of holistic care are covered, including clinical skills and relevant social/life sciences. It contains activities, two-colour illustrations and a website with MCQs and much more. Well worth buying.

Ethics

Rumbold, G., 2000. Ethics in Nursing Practice, third edn. Baillière Tindall, Edinburgh
Easy to read, presented plainly and in clear language, this book discusses relationships with patients and other professionals, and the way ethics impact on decisions nurses make. A classic book and a real 'must have'.

Health promotion

Naidoo, J., Wills, J., 2000. Health Promotion, second edn. Baillière Tindall, London
An excellent basic health promotion text, this outlines everything from how to assess a community's health to strategies to improve health and evaluate the effectiveness of those strategies. It is clear and plainly written. Useful in community nursing modules.

Leadership

www.nursingleadership.org.uk
The Foundation of Nursing Leadership. A collection of free nursing leadership resources.

Learning styles

Hinchliff, S., Eaton, A., Howard, S., Thompson, S., 2003. Practitioner as Teacher, third edn. Churchill Livingstone, Edinburgh
This book is really intended for qualified nurses who want to be a mentor or teacher, but it's a good resource for a student nurse too. It discusses the way people learn and learning in the clinical environment. Light, clear and easy to read, it lets you in on what your mentors and teachers are trying to do!

Legal issues

Dimond, B., 2008. Legal Aspects of Nursing, fifth edn. Prentice-Hall, London
I don't know this book well, but it comes very highly recommended as the best general book about legal issues in nursing.

Models and theories

If you become very interested in a specific model, you can look for additional information by that specific nursing theorist in your library.

Pearson, A., Vaughn, B., Fitzgerald, M., 2005. **Nursing Models for Practice, third edn. Butterworth-Heinemann, Oxford**
Easy to read and understand, very clear and, although not really comprehensive, should give you everything that you need.

Nursing practice

Hinchliff, S., Norman, S., Schober, J., 2008. **Nursing Practice and Health Care: A Foundation Text, fifth edn. Edward Arnold, London**
A clearly written book that explains elements of care in common foundation and in each of the different branches. It is great for helping you learn to think and behave as a nurse. An excellent resource for assignments as well.

Walsh, M., (ed) 2007. **Watson's Clinical Nursing and Related Sciences, seventh edn. Baillière Tindall, Edinburgh**
Approaches patient care system by system, and is comprehensive but easy to read. A good investment as it discusses not only the nursing care, but also the related anatomy and physiology. Great to use for preparing for placements, and will be useful after your course.

Research

Craig, J., Smyth, R., 2007. **The Evidence-Based Practice Manual for Nurses. Churchill Livingstone, Edinburgh**
Most of this is a little advanced for a brand new student, but it has an absolutely brilliant section on how to do a literature search and is worth buying just for that chapter. Has an impressive list of resources to help you search.

Lanoe, N., 2002. **Ogier's Reading Research: How to Make Research More Approachable, third edn. Baillière Tindall, London**
Good book that will guide you through reading and thinking about research, although it won't really help you write research.

Parahoo, K., 2006. **Nursing Research: Principles, Process and Issues, second edn. Macmillan, Basingstoke**
A great book that can help you understand or actually do research. Clearly written with good examples and explanations.

Reflection

There is a lot available online and in journals about reflection, and reflection is mentioned in nursing texts about many other subjects. The Maslin-Prothero book in the study skills section is very good on reflection. If you do decide to buy a book, look at the two below, or find something that you can relate to by looking at reflective practice books in the nursing library before buying one.

Johns, C., 2009. Becoming a Reflective Practitioner: A Reflective and Holistic Approach to Clinical Nursing, Practice Development and Clinical Supervision, third edn. Wiley-Blackwell, Oxford
Johns, C., Freshwater, D., (eds) 2005. Transforming Nursing Through Reflective Practice, second edn. Wiley-Blackwell, Oxford

Social policy

Although a good book can help you understand the background to current policy, social policy changes faster than any textbook can follow. For the most current details, look at the Department of Health and NHS websites (always read the executive summary before wading through any government document).

Ham, C., 2004. Health Policy in Britain: The Politics and Organization of the National Health Service, fifth edn. Macmillan, Basingstoke
This book is pretty easy to read, considering the subject matter, and helps you understand not just about where policy has come from but also why it evolved the way it did.

www.dh.gov.uk
www.nhs.uk

You can look at national sites as well:

www.scot.nhs.uk
www.scotland.gov.uk
www.wales.nhs.uk
www.dhsspsni.gov.uk
www.n-i.nhs.uk

Study skills

Goodall, C., 1995. A Survivor's Guide to Study Skills and Student Assessments. Churchill Livingstone, Edinburgh
A basic book, light to read, but very useful.

Maslin-Prothero, S., (ed) 2001. Baillière's Study Skills for Nurses, second edn. Baillière Tindall, London
A good basic all-round book, very thorough and easy to read. If you only get one study skills book, get this one.

Taylor, J., 2001. Baillière's Study Skills for Nurses. Baillière Tindall, London
A small, older book, but has good hints and tips about presentations and seminars among other things.

MAGAZINES AND JOURNALS

For CFP students, the *Nursing Standard* (*NS*) and the *Nursing Times* (*NT*) are great reading and have special rates for students. You can also access them online through your university's library resources. These are great gifts to ask your family for. Search for 'Nursing Standard' or 'Nursing Times' online to access their home pages. If you buy one copy (which they will have in your university's shop or at any hospital newsagent), there is information inside on how to subscribe.

There are other journals. The *British Journal of Nursing* (*BJN*) is great, but might be a little advanced for a new student. Wait until you are at the end of your second or beginning of your third year to get this journal, to make sure you are up to it.

The publishers of the *NS*, *NT* and *BNJ* put out some specialty journals. You might be able to get a discount, but this is not offered on all of them.

There are many nursing magazines from the USA, but be careful, because standards of practice and care systems are very different and the material might not fit in with your role as a nurse in the UK.

Appendix 1
The National Union of Students – NUS

You might encounter two types of 'student union' while you are a student. There is the National Union of Students (NUS) – an organization that supports students in many different capacities across the UK (there are NUS branches in each of the four UK countries) – and unions of students that are not affiliated with the NUS. Even if your local office is not specifically affiliated with the NUS, it will still offer support and help. You can get a lot of information about the NUS quite easily:

- Pop into the NUS office on your campus (the best way)
- Go to www.nus.org.uk (the next best way)
- Call your university switchboard and ask to speak to the Union of Students office (from personal experience, some receptionists will not be very well informed or will be very busy – it's better to go in person or check the web!).

What does the NUS offer you?

- Your NUS card, which entitles you to many different student discounts and is accepted as proof of your student status in most places
- Information about benefits and discounts for students
- Support for international students
- Help with government forms, such as entitlement to free prescriptions
- Documents about student issues, such as housing and finances
- Publications about every aspect of university and student life
- Advice from advisors trained to support students who are having academic, personal or financial problems
- Help in planning events, such us a student ball or other student activity
- Help in joining a union or any student group/organization
- The NUS usually runs a shop for students, and often runs a bar as well
- Activities and fun events on campus
- Representation in academic (but not clinical placement related) disciplinary proceedings and cheating boards

- A university newsletter or newspaper
- Fresher's fairs
- Advocacy for national student issues – the NUS sends representatives to political party conferences, meets with governmental officials, and has advisors and elected officials working actively to promote student welfare through government support and policy.

In addition, if you are a group rep, or steward/representative for Unison, the Royal College of Nursing (RCN) or the Royal College of Midwives (RCM), the NUS office can often offer you some office space and support for official duties.

Your university gives the NUS funding based on student numbers (it's usually £1 or less per head). Sadly, some campuses or satellites that have mainly or all nursing students have a history of not being as well supported as the campuses that have 'traditional' students (you know, the recent school leavers who attend classes Monday to Friday, 9 am to 3.30 pm, and who have regular holidays and the summer off), so if you need help, speak up. The NUS is usually very good at adapting to meeting students' needs. You can also run for local, regional or national office in the NUS.

In addition to supporting students, the NUS represents the student viewpoint by organizing and participating in demonstrations, lobbying government, and raising money for local and national charities.

However, there are a few problems for the NUS in helping nursing students: first, the influx of large numbers of nursing students has perhaps overwhelmed the NUS a bit; second, the emergence of satellite campuses devoted to nursing but without (usually) student residences and university offices (the usual locations for NUS offices); and third, the schedules for nursing courses (throughout the summer, in the evening and even some weekends); they all have made it difficult for the NUS to keep up with the demand for services. At this time, the NUS doesn't have the resources or information to help student nurses with problems related specifically to clinical placements. However, it has identified many of these issues as problems that must be addressed, and is trying to put in place national-level representatives whose role it is to look into and support the types of problems student nurses have – both as a result of their course and in accessing NUS services.

What should you go to the NUS for? Not all NUS offices will offer everything – if you need something, just call or drop in and ask:

- Academic problems: when you think something is unfair, when you think the university has violated a policy or correct procedure, when you have been accused of an academic offence like cheating, or when you need help with academic skills. The NUS will also support your group reps (students elected in each cohort to represent student perspectives on university governance groups and to raise concerns and issues).

- Complaints: you can raise complaints and concerns about the university, campus, university housing, etc., through the NUS.
- Personal problems: relationship problems, physical health issues, bullying, mental health, issues related to sexuality and sexual health, financial problems, disabilities, problems or questions about housing, etc. They also offer advice on crime prevention and safety, and you can usually get an inexpensive personal alarm through the NUS.
- Lifestyle: information about discounts, the local nightlife, events, student-friendly businesses, part-time work, support for international students, etc. The NUS has career information (not a lot of it is great for nurses, but they are improving this), and can give advice and guidance about CVs and interviews.
- Activities: the NUS office will have information on clubs, sports, organizations and groups on campus. They also will support you if you want to plan a trip, event or activity such as a graduation ball (hint: you need at least a year to plan a graduation ball, in part because of placements, but also because it takes a lot of time – go see them sooner rather than later!)
- Other resources: the NUS will be able to point you in the direction of someone who can help you if they can't. They will have many valuable publications from the NUS, from the university and from other organizations.
- Fax and photocopy services.

The NUS is an excellent organization that offers support and assistance in nearly every type of query or problem you may have. It does not, however, offer any support or assistance if your problem is related to clinical placements. You are still likely to need help and support from one of the unions that support nursing students (Unison, the RCN or the RCM). Each of these organizations has special resources and information targeted specifically for nursing (or midwifery) students.

Go and visit your student union office; get your NUS card; see what's on offer and if you have a little time or some expertise in a particular area, offer to help. The NUS is for students, by students . . . it can always use your help and support.

Appendix 2
Nursing and Midwifery Council (NMC) Standards for Pre-Registration Nursing Education (2010)

INTRODUCTION

The NMC *Standards for Pre-Registration Nursing Education*, published in 2010, ensures that all graduate nursing education (from 2013) will be responsive to 'changing needs, developments, priorities and expectations in health and healthcare'. Those nurses who meet the standards 'will be equipped to meet these present and future challenges, improve health and wellbeing and drive up standards and quality, working in a range of roles including practitioner, educator, leader and researcher' (NMC 2010, p.4).

FIELDS

There are four specific fields of nursing:

- Adult nursing
- Mental health nursing
- Children's nursing
- Learning disabilities nursing.

STANDARDS FOR COMPETENCE

The competency framework sets out the competencies that every nursing student must attain before they can become a registered nurse. Each of the four fields (see above) has separate competency requirements, and these are listed under four domains. These are:

- Professional values
- Communication and interpersonal skills
- Nursing practice and decision-making
- Leadership, management and team working.

'Each domain is comprised of a generic standard for competence and a field standard for competence. It also includes the generic competencies that all nurses must achieve and the field competencies to be achieved in each specific field' (NMC 2010, p.11).

ESSENTIAL SKILLS CLUSTERS (ESCs)

The five essential skills clusters are:

- Care, compassion and communication
- Organizational aspects of care
- Infection prevention and control
- Nutrition and fluid management
- Medicines management.

There are three progression points – first progression point, second progression point, and entry to the register; however, skills have not been identified for all three progression points.

Note: Chapter 1, Becoming and being a Nurse, provides further information about new pre-registration standards.

REFERENCE

Nursing Midwifery Council (NMC), 2010. Standards for Pre-Registration Nursing Education. NMC, London.

There is a lot in the news about people with mental health problems being a danger to society. There has been uproar from the public asking for dangerous people to be put 'away', far from those of us who fear them; those of us who are frightened by people who talk to themselves, who hear voices, and who imagine that others are out to get them.

Is this all there is to mental health problems? Are people with mental health problems all a dangerous lot against whom we need defence, locking them away, forcing them to take medication they don't want in order to prevent them from becoming evil killers without a conscience?

Granted, a few people with some serious mental health problems are dangerous, but by a long margin, most of them are just like you and me – because they *are* you and me. Up to 85 per cent of the population suffers from a mental health problem at some point in time. Nurses who care for those with mental health problems are experts at diagnosing the problem and helping people to come to an understanding of their problem, themselves, the treatment they need and the help they require to live fruitful lives. For some people this will mean a return to a 'normal' life, but others will need a lifetime of care and support. At every place people with mental health problems go on their life journey, there will be a mental health nurse there to support them.

Mental health nurses work in forensics (prisons and hospitals for the mentally ill who are court ordered into custody), in general hospitals, in the community, visiting people in homes or seeing them in clinics… they work with families, children, adolescents, adults, older adults… across the board.

As a mental health nurse, there are some key things you need to remember:

1. Mental health impacts on physical health, and physical health impacts on mental health.
2. Just because someone has a mental health problem it doesn't mean they can't give (or deny) consent. Most people with mental health problems lead independent lives and are able to make the correct decisions

for themselves; however, some people may lack this capacity. You need to know the Mental Capacity Act (MCA 2005) inside out to make sure you apply the law properly.

3. Never, ever be untruthful. Once you have lost trust, you have nothing to work with. Never tell a client that you will keep a secret. You can't help them if you aren't honest.

4. There's a saying: 'Just because you're paranoid doesn't mean that someone isn't out to get you!' Remember that no matter what a person's problem is, you still must take their complaints seriously. Don't just assume that someone complaining of pain or other symptoms is exhibiting attention-seeking behaviour.

5. Sensible boundaries are essential. You need to be aware of emotional and physical boundaries; someone with a mental health problem may misinterpret actions or comments you make. Be careful so you can continue to be therapeutic for your clients. Don't dress in a way that could upset your clients: football strips, clothes with logos or political/religious symbols or that could be considered revealing/provocative could all upset clients with mental health problems. Dress in a neutral, professional way. Also be aware as well that some clients could react to your size, racial group, shape, hair colour, body jewellery, tattoos, etc.

6. Some people with mental health problems can be very manipulative or charismatic. Be cautious and always be objective. Always leave yourself a way out of a situation – never allow a client to get between you and an exit. You can't help people if you don't keep yourself safe.

7. Some people will never get any better, and for some people what appear to be insignificant achievements are major triumphs. Praise your clients for their hard work.

8. As a student, you should *never* provide one-to-one supervision for a client. You yourself need supervision, so how can you supervise anyone else?

9. A person is not their diagnosis. Just because there are many common characteristics in a disease doesn't mean any person is a 'typical manic' or a 'typical schizophrenic'. See your clients as individuals, and don't fall into the habit of seeing people only as their diagnosis.

10. Many nurses in all different fields and areas suffer from stress and stress-related problems. Don't try to cure yourself through your job. You are there to be therapeutic for your clients, not for them to help you.

Many people with mental health problems become manipulative – not because they are bad people (no one is a 'bad person' because of mental health issues, even though they might do 'bad' things), but because it's the best way they have found to get their needs met. We all use our strengths – and, for some, manipulative behaviour is a strength. For this reason it is essential for you to protect yourself (and your client) by being very careful, and not doing anything that you know you shouldn't. One slip and your rapport with your patient could be lost.

A few people with mental health problems may have different ideas about hygiene and personal care to that of society – they may not wash often enough, they may have body odour, they may not want to change clothes. At times, not washing or changing clothes may be a challenge to the mental health staff: 'Look, I am not following the rules, what are you going to do about it?' For some, failures in hygiene are because they don't have the energy or focus to do things for themselves. For others, they care so little about themselves that they don't want to care about things like clean clothes or showering. For very few, they see their lack of hygiene as protection from a world that is out to get them. Help, encourage and offer support, but try not to be too critical of people who struggle to be clean – you will in time learn the difference between people who need sympathy and help, and those who need to be told to stop playing games and grab a flannel.

Many people with mental health problems misuse other drugs, including alcohol – some legal, some not. This is not because there is a tendency for people to be drug users; it's because they have emotional pain and are looking for help to stop the pain. Being drunk or high helps in the short term, even though it may make the long term much worse. Don't be judgemental.

Caring for your own hygiene and appearance is only one part of self-care. People with mental health problems might not eat properly, might get too little (or too much) sleep, might not visit the dentist, etc. Looking at the Essence of Care document (DH, 2010), you have all the basics you need to help someone care for themselves. Don't think that as a mental health nurse you only have to worry about the patient's mind – you have to see them and care for them as a whole person and meet their most basic needs, even if the most important thing for them is washing their hair.

As a student nurse, don't get hurt. Don't feel pity for the clients. Always treat them with dignity and respect. They have a valid condition; one which causes them physical, psychological, emotional and spiritual pain. The clients may make poor decisions or commit criminal acts; separate the condition from the person, and always try to see good even in the most difficult of clients. Don't fool yourself; keep your appraisal honest and be realistic about the risks you face, but at least be willing to see the good beneath the damage done by the condition. For many, a mental health problem is similar to a cancer that destroys and scars the most central parts of a personality; too often, we judge the person by the 'cancer' instead of everything else.

Finally, promote mental health awareness wherever you go. Help reduce the stigma by telling people the reality – that a mental health problem is not a character flaw, it is not the lack of a soul, it is rarely incurable and it does not make monsters of those ill with it. People with mental health problems are entitled to the same respect, dignity and care as those with a physical condition such as diabetes, cancer or heart disease. That dignity and respect starts with you.

REFERENCES

Department of Health (DH), 2010. Essence of Care 2010. TSO, Norwich; www.dh.gov.uk/en/Publicationsandstatistics/Publications/Publications PolicyAndGuidance/DH_119969, accessed August 2012

Department for Constitutionals Affairs, 2007. Mental Capacity Act 2005. Code of Practice. TSO, Norwich; www.legislation.gov.uk/ukpga/2005/9/contents, accessed November 2012

Appendix 4
Learning Disabilities Nursing
Denise Stevens

One of the first things I wanted to learn as a student nurse in learning disability nursing was: what do registered nurses actually do? I was several months into my nursing course at university before my first practical placement and I actually had no idea of what nurses in this field did. I very excitedly asked my fellow students who had previously worked as support staff in residential homes for adults with learning disabilities, only to discover that everyone appeared to have their own ideas of what constituted a registered nurse in learning disabilities nursing (RNLD). One student even suggested that learning disability nurses spent their days travelling around weighing clients!

HISTORY

The historical 'care' or 'treatment' of learning disabled people has had an enormous impact on the current role of today's RNLD. For example, as long ago as the fifteenth century, people with a learning disability were stigmatized and considered to be lunatics. Treatment consisted of being chained and whipped (Gates 1997). In the sixteenth century, learning disabilities were linked to witchcraft and learning disabled people were locked away, often with keepers they feared. In the eighteenth and nineteenth centuries, those considered to be 'lunatics' were separated from paupers. Aristocratic patients often lived in private asylums that provided accommodation of a similar level of comfort to that found in upper-class family homes (Scull 1979), but, despite the surroundings, few improved and the private asylums were in fact just luxurious prisons. In comparison, the private madhouses that housed pauper 'lunatics' were described as desperately cruel, and conditions were abominable (Scull 1979). Treatment consisted of bleeding, the drug digitalis, electricity and emetics (Gates 1997). Many patients were kept in irons; there were no baths, books or employment, and there was often only one staff member to as many as 50 patients. Reforms brought in in the nineteenth century were initially intended to cure patients, but with the low cure rates, the emphasis changed to providing more humane living conditions, such as clean bedding, sufficient clothing, an absence of chains, and regular attendance at church. In the mid-twentieth century, Nazi Germany exterminated people with a mental handicap, along with others they considered to be undesirable.

It was not until the 1970s that conditions for people with learning disabilities finally began to improve, after damaging publicity regarding the ill treatment and substandard living conditions in large institutions. Patients often had no personal possessions, clothing or space (Swann 1997). Barton (1960) identified a separate condition, known as 'institutional neurosis', which resulted from the institutionalized care received by people with learning disabilities in mental hospitals. The condition was characterized by apathy, lack of initiative or interest, submissiveness, deterioration in personal habits, and resignation to their surroundings. The White Paper *Better Services for the Mentally Handicapped* was published in 1971, but it was not until 1990 that the NHS and Community Care Act became law.

THE PRESENT DAY

The implementation of the 1990 Act was the beginning of the slow move from institutional care to improved community care. The care of people with learning disabilities has evolved over the centuries, with the most dramatic changes occurring since the 1970s with the concept of de-institutionalization and normalization.

The concept of normalization was developed as long ago as 1959 in Denmark and 1969 in Sweden (Swann 1997). Wolfensberger (1972) states that normalization seeks to value client groups who were previously devalued. To do this, Wolfensberger (1972) promoted social role valorization and believed that people with learning disabilities needed to be seen to be leading socially valued lives by living as part of the community, accessing local facilities, and having the same rights and opportunities as everyone else. Many trusts now use the John O'Brien 'five service accomplishments' as a method of implementing the concept of normalization into care delivery. This is considered to be a 'user-friendly' approach that gives a set of values together with a framework for use (Plougher 1997).

It is these basic philosophies of normalization and social role valorization that underpin the work of the nurse in learning disabilities and service provision. In response to the considerable changes in the care of people with learning disabilities and to de-institutionalization, the role of the nurse in learning disabilities has also had to adapt and evolve, and is continuing to do so.

Fortunately, the role of the nurse in learning disabilities is no longer deciding which chains to use, and working in this service is now extremely rewarding. It is now possible to play an important role in facilitating people to be as independent as possible and to have real choices over their own lives.

THE ROLE OF THE LEARNING DISABILITY NURSE

There would appear to be many views on the role of the learning disabilities nurse. According to Baldwin and Birchenall (Gates 1997), there are six key roles: clinician, counsellor, advisor/advocate, manager, educator and therapist. As with all branches of nursing, the nursing intervention depends on the needs of the individual. For example, a person with a mild learning disability may be able to live independently, be in employment and only need nursing intervention for reasons such as administration of medication, dietary advice or monitoring. A person with a profound learning disability may also be physically disabled with no sensory, communication or learning ability, and be completely dependent on carers for all of his or her personal and health needs. There are also some people with learning disabilities who present with severe behavioural problems that require specialist knowledge and skills. These behaviours can also vary, from people with poor social skills or inappropriate sexual behaviour, to those who exhibit aggressive, threatening or self-injurious behaviour. There are also learning disability nurses working in the forensic service with offenders – for example, sex offenders and firesetters. These varied roles are unique to the RNLD. According to Butler (2003), skills such as 'high level social development and behavioural knowledge' (p. 28) are what make learning disability nurses so highly valued. It must also be remembered that people with learning disabilities have the same health problems as the rest of society, as well as the unique health issues of those with genetic disorders and syndromes.

Life in learning disability nursing can also be extremely interesting, providing the setting for many anecdotal stories. For example ...

On one occasion a young, male client was staring quite intently. When asked if he was all right, he shook his head to indicate that he was not. He was asked if he wanted something, to which he nodded his head to indicate 'yes'. When asked what he would like his answer can only be described as 'personal services'! I had to explain to him that this was not in my remit as a student nurse, I was unable to oblige, and he was offered a cup of tea instead!

Always read client care plans

Because of the very diverse client groups within the learning disability service, each with their unique needs, the 'top tips' to students are also very client specific. However, there is some advice that may be useful to all student nurses in learning disabilities. For example, always read client care plans as soon as possible when on placement. There may be clients who exhibit challenging behaviours and have behavioural programmes in place; the care plans will give information as to triggers to the behaviours and advice on how to manage them. It is only when everyone who is involved with the client works consistently that behavioural programmes can be successful in reducing unwanted behaviours. It can take only one person to seriously undermine and jeopardize success. Reading client care plans will inform you of any client allergies, preferences or dislikes. An example of this is that many learning disabled adults have been subject to abuse, whether physical, sexual, psychological or financial. A client who has suffered previous abuse may not like a particular gender to be involved in his or her personal care. He or she may not like physical touch and might react quite strongly when touched, even accidentally. It is also important to remember that any new face on a unit, even a well-intentioned student, can be very unsettling for a person with a learning disability. It can take time to earn the trust and confidence of a client, so taking the time to get to know someone before being involved in his or her personal care is good practice.

Always read trust policies

It is important also to read local trust policies and procedures, together with any specific unit policies. Student nurses must work in accordance with trust policies. It cannot be assumed that all staff work in accordance with these policies, but by being informed of expected practices a student nurse can avoid being compromised.

BEING A STUDENT NURSE

Every student nurse should be aware of the Nursing and Midwifery Council (NMC) guidelines for student nurses (2010). Students are sometimes asked to carry out duties that are inappropriate and unacceptable, and this can seriously risk patient safety. For example, one first-year student nurse on her first practical placement was asked to perform male urinary catheterization and, although this request was from a very insistent doctor, she had the good sense to refuse. A second-year student nurse was asked to administer client medication in a nursing home environment without the supervision of qualified or drug-assessed staff, and she was encouraged to take sole responsibility for this duty. Drug errors are all too easy to make for even the most diligent of qualified nurses, and can be potentially fatal, so it is understandable that the administration of medicines by unsupervised student nurses is against all guidelines and policies. Medication charts in learning disability premises often have an accompanying photograph of the client to aid recognition – extremely useful when being asked to administer medication in an unfamiliar environment.

The open culture in nursing now encourages disclosure of mistakes as a learning tool for others. A nurse is no longer disciplined for medication errors, but *will* be disciplined for not following procedure. If an error occurs, be honest and ensure the correct care for the client; do not try to cover it up because this is professional suicide and clearly unethical and not in the client's best interest. Several fellow students have been asked to lift clients physically without the use of hoisting equipment, this being accepted practice by regular staff despite there being 'no lifting' policies. The students felt isolated when taking a stand against lifting clients, but nurses and student nurses alike need to advocate good, safe and legal practice. Also, if a student nurse is injured when physically lifting a client, she will not be insured!

Occasional 'pockets' of staff do not adhere to the philosophy of normalization and do not work with learning disabled clients in a respectful or dignified way. It can be difficult for a student nurse to flag up problem areas or concerns when on practical placement, and she may have difficult choices to make, especially given the need to pass placements. But whistle-blowing creates dilemmas for both student and qualified nurses alike. One senior nurse advised that when in a difficult situation, it might help to visualize it on the front page of a newspaper – how would it look? Can you justify your action or lack of action? Always remember the network of student support that is available, such as university lecturers and placement coordinators, trust staff, mentors and managers, and peer group support and telephone advice lines run by the NMC and RCN. There is a wealth of experienced people who will be only too happy to offer support and advice. Sometimes it just feels better to talk to someone and air our feelings.

As learning disability nurses do not wear a uniform, it is a good idea to wear clothes that are loose, comfortable and laundry-friendly. Trousers and blouses may need to be washed several times a week. One colleague was recently in the wrong place at the wrong time when a client was suffering from projectile vomiting (perhaps this is not the time to mention the diarrhoea he was also suffering from!), so it can also be prudent to have a spare set of clothes nearby, working on the assumption that if you do not have any you will definitely need them! It is probably also a good idea to leave the designer gear at home.

The forensic service

If as a student nurse you are fortunate to be offered the opportunity of a placement in the forensic service, there are some basic guidelines. These include reading unit policies and client care plans – it is important to remember that these clients are offenders and should not be underestimated, however inoffensive or likeable they appear. The wearing of suitable clothes is essential, and can be discussed before beginning the placement. No personal information should be discussed with clients or within earshot of clients. This includes any information regarding family members or addresses, and especially photographs. Offenders, particularly sex offenders, can be very manipulative and use the information for their own benefit. Physical contact between fellow staff or clients is also seriously discouraged; this includes hugs and kisses at the end of the placement! Providing the unit advice is followed, the placement should be fascinating and a superb learning opportunity.

Helpful books and resources

Useful reading simply has to include *Learning Disabilities: Towards Inclusion* (edited by Atherton and Crickmore). This book, which is the sixth edition of *Learning Disabilities*, formerly edited by Gates and cited above, has a contemporary approach reflecting practice developments, including the impact on services of changing policy and legislation.

The A–Z of Syndromes and Inherited Disorders by Gilbert is an excellent reference book of conditions for nurses in all fields. The White Paper *Valuing People* by the Department of Health sets government targets and planning for people with a learning disability. The Mental Health Act 2007 is useful when working with clients who are held under a section of the Act (although relevant sections may be preferable to the entire Act!). *The Psychology of Criminal Conduct* by Blackburn is a fascinating read when working in forensic nursing. The Human Rights Act (1998) is also useful for clients' basic rights. *Nursing Law and Ethics* by Tingle and Cribb is an excellent book for students of all fields. Details of all these (and other) resources are in the References section at the end of this appendix. Finally, a good nursing dictionary is a must! Another good tip is to buy books that will also be of use to you after qualifying.

Becoming qualified

Perhaps the most important advice is to believe in your ability to complete the nursing course. The high drop-out rate of student nurses, together with the fact that many mature students have not studied academically for several years, can be very daunting. Younger students have the advantage of being more recently in the education system, perhaps studying subjects useful to nursing, such as the sciences, but mature students have the advantage of life experience and time-management skills. These different skills are equally important, and can be very levelling. From experience, it is not always the brightest students who pass modules, but those who have the commitment and determination to succeed and work diligently. The course is a 3-year marathon and not a quick sprint! There are always some students on the course who gain impressive marks when revising for an exam or writing an assignment only days before the submission date, only to become complacent and fail modules at a later date. From experience, these are often the students who later struggle to complete the course, because underestimated course modules mounted up. Take time and effort to work studiously, prepare and revise while the subject is still fresh in your mind, but only do it once! Try to avoid re-sitting exams or having to re-submit assignments several months after the original deadline.

To some students, the thought of being organized is a very unpleasant one. Be organized in writing assignments; even if you work better under pressure and prefer to write assignments close to the submission date, you can carry out research and identify articles needed in advance. For those who, like the writer, are technophobes and believe that computers have the ability to plan and sabotage work, please remember that computers only crash or run out of ink on the eve of a deadline. This behaviour is almost unheard of with a month to go!

One student was heard to complain that she very unfairly had three assignment deadlines within 3 days of each other. However, when she was reminded that the assignments had all been launched 6 or 7 months previously, she simply answered 'That's not the point'. Being organized, although it is a very boring concept, also allows for the unexpected, such as a bout of 'flu or unexpected family commitments. One piece of advice from a lecturer was to type an assignment and 'let it go cold' for a few days, after which it can be proofread objectively and the writer does not read what he or she expects to read.

Never be embarrassed to ask questions in lectures. Many students are just too self-conscious to ask a question or admit they don't understand something in front of so many other people. However, one thing for certain is that there will be many other people who don't know the answer either and are waiting patiently for someone else to ask.

Take advantage of all learning opportunities. The advantages of attending extra sessions, such as academic writing groups, skills practice or a day with a paramedic, far outweigh having a little extra time off. The 3-year training period is also an ideal opportunity to request placements with different health trusts and in specialist areas, enabling student nurses to have an overview of how different trusts work. This can also be an opportunity to network, make valuable friendships and learn about career opportunities.

Finally, perhaps the most important and valuable piece of advice any student nurse can have: simply enjoy the entire experience!

REFERENCES AND BIBLIOGRAPHY

Atherton, H.L., Crickmore, D., (eds.) 2011. Learning Disabilities: Toward Inclusion, sixth ed. Churchill Livingstone, Edinburgh

Barton, R., 1960. Institutional neurosis. Reprinted in: Gates, B., (ed.) 1997. Learning Disabilities, third ed. Churchill Livingstone, Edinburgh

Blackburn, R., 1995. The Psychology of Criminal Conduct. Wiley-Blackwell, Oxford

Butler, B., 2003. Nursing in the 21st Century. Learning Disability Practice 6(2): 28

Craft, A., 1994. Practice Issues in Sexuality and Learning Disabilities. Routledge, London

Department of Health (DH), 1990. NHS and Community Care Act 1990. www.legislation.gov.uk/ukpga/1990/19/contents; accessed November 2012

Department of Health (DH), 1998. Signposts for Success in Commissioning and Providing Health Services for People with Learning Disabilities. NHS Executive, Leeds

Department of Health (DH), 2001. Valuing People: A New Strategy for Learning Disability for the 21st Century. The Stationery Office, London

Department of Health (DH), 2007. Mental Health Act 2007. DH, London; www.legislation.gov.uk/ukpga/2007/12/contents; accessed January 2013

Gates, B., (ed.) 1997. Learning Disabilities, third ed. Churchill Livingstone, New York

Gilbert, P., 2000. A–Z of Syndromes and Inherited Disorders, third ed. Stanley Thornes, Cheltenham

Nursing and Midwifery Council (NMC), 2010. Guidance on Professional Conduct for Nursing and Midwifery Students, second ed. www.nmc-uk.org/Documents/Guidance/NMC-Guidance-on-professional-conduct-for-nursing-and-midwifery-students.pdf; accessed November 2012

Plougher, J., 1997. Providing quality care. In: Gates, B., (ed.) 1997. Learning Disabilities. Churchill Livingstone, New York, NY

Scull, A. T., 1982. Museums of Madness. Penguin, Harmondsworth, Middlesex

Swann, C., 1997. Development of services. In: Gates, B., (ed.) 1997. Learning Disabilities. Churchill Livingstone, New York

Tingle, J., Cribb, A., (eds.) 2007. Nursing Law and Ethics, third ed. Blackwell Science, Oxford

United Nations, 1971. Declaration of Rights of Mentally Retarded Persons. United Nations, New York

Wolfensburge, W., 1972. Cited in Stalker, K., Campbell, V., 1998. Person-centred planning: An evaluation of a training programme. Health and Social Care in the Community 6(2): 130–134

WEBSITES

Choice Support: www.choicesupport.org.uk

Mencap: www.mencap.org.uk

Nursing and Midwifery Council: www.nmc-uk.org

Appendix 5
Tips for Children's Nursing

I saw a sign in a book on nursing history: it said 'Parents may visit Children on the second and fourth Thursdays of the month, from 2.15 until 2.45, or 4.15–4.45, at the Matron's discretion'. The sign was next to a gallery – it was obvious that the parents stood outside, and the children were brought to the gallery. There was a grille between where the parents stood and where their children would be. Imagine – your child is ill, maybe dying, and you are allowed to see them for half an hour, every 2 weeks, but not allowed even to touch them ... is that good care by today's standards? It was the norm then.

I saw, in the same book, the results of an essay contest by young patients on that ward. They spoke about how they made toys, how they helped care for other patients, and one spoke about how she helped to make bandages ... it showed this child to be very busy, not doing things we associate with being in a hospital, but more things just to keep busy.

Children's nursing has progressed tremendously since this time so many years ago; we have developed an understanding that children are not miniature adults but special people with specific needs, and their developmental processes must be recognized to allow them to develop normally even though they may be in hospital or in care for prolonged periods of time.

Children react very quickly; they decide who to trust and who to be afraid of, and once they make this decision it is nearly impossible to change. The physical processes are as mercurial as their emotional changes – a child's condition can change very quickly and, as a result, they can become seriously ill in a fraction of the time it would take an adult. For this reason children require special monitoring and attentiveness, an individual with special training in the needs and their health: the children's nurse.

You don't need to ask children who are most important in their life, you just need to look at the way they cling to their mother, father or other loved one as they are carried into the hospital or into the surgery. Failing to involve the parents or guardians in a child's care means taking away the support they need to make decisions and to feel secure in whatever happens to them. Although at any age a child has a right to consent to some degree, it is usually the parents or guardian who are required to make decisions about consent. If they have not been involved and don't understand what is happening to the child, then they will not be able to make the best and most informed decision.

Children have keen survival skills: they learn very quickly – and make a judgement even more quickly – about the people around them. If you lie to a child even about something small, you have completely destroyed trust; that child will not forget, and there will be little you can do in the future to get them to trust you again. Even though parents or guardians are required to give consent at most times, remember that gaining the child's cooperation and engagement is the ideal. It is easier to do something with the child's cooperation than to inflict and suffer the trauma resulting from a screaming, kicking and fighting child who will do anything in his or her power to escape the people trying to help; this is difficult not only for the child but also for the parents, the other children in the care environment, and every single member of staff. Getting a child to work with you is the only way to do your job properly. Children are insightful and have a way of knowing things you don't expect them to. They might not tell you they know because they are trying to protect *you*! Honest communication is important, but never lead anyone to lose hope.

You need to love the children you care for, but you can't compromise your objectivity and professionalism. Speak at the appropriate level. Use words a child can understand even if it seems silly. Asking children if they have opened their bowels may be confusing – it's better to say, 'Did you poo?' Remember that they will see you as an adult in authority and might need to be given permission to ask questions or express their concerns. It also helps to know what trends are current in children's TV and books so you have something to talk about! Children use a lot of non-verbal communication. When caring for children, you need to be sensitive to what they *don't* say, and how they behave. Just because a child is quiet or sleeping doesn't mean he or she isn't in pain or very ill. Don't take anything for granted.

Medication administration is very specific in children's nursing. Have the necessary formulas and titrations written down and always use them. Children have what is called a 'paradoxical reaction' to many medications; this means that what can make an adult tired can make a child hyperactive, and *vice versa*! Always know what the medication you are giving will do to a *child*. Although children might not have understanding of pharmacological principles, it's still important to try to help them understand why they are taking medicines.

As a children's nurse you will have heartache and tears, but you will also have joy and satisfaction. Take care of yourself: you can't take care of anyone else if you don't take care of yourself.

Thanks to Elaine Elswell for her contributions to this section.

Nursing Older People

Older people comprise one of the most vulnerable groups in healthcare today: the news is full of reports showing that older people are not receiving the care they require. Many nursing students feel that care of the older person is all about incontinence, manual handling and dementia: this is the stereotype, but it is a fair one. Many older people may require assistance that younger people do not, but this does not mean that all older people are sitting in rise-and-recline chairs, with wet underwear and no awareness of who or where they are. Most older people lead active lives that are only occasionally marred by illness. Although older adults are defined as those aged 65 years or over, it is important to remember that many people continue in paid work long after 65, and a significant number of older people manage well into their 80s and beyond.

The care of the older person is steeped in the best nursing can offer: excellent assessment and skilled personal care will give an older person help to regain lost independence; insight into the needs of older people and their developmental stages (it's not just children who are developing) guides the older person's nurse into making decisions that lead patients to health and a fulfilling life, even though health might not mean being free from illness.

Health promotion and health education are especially rewarding for older people, as some may tend to believe that there is nothing new to learn: being given the opportunity to learn new things is not only fun, but can contribute to improved health.

The older person often has to deal with more loss than someone younger: loss of independence, loss of health, loss of sensory input from poor vision or poor hearing, and bereavement. Close friends, family members or a loved partner are all also growing older, and loss not only causes pain but is also a reminder that older person too is heading towards the end of his or her life. A nurse can compassionately help patients to grieve and prepare for their own death, and assist them in maintaining loving memories of those who have died. This is especially important when the individual suffers from cognitive losses, such as dementia.

All in all, although care of the older person can be demanding and heavy work, it is also rewarding and enjoyable. The patients have a sense of history and perspective that one cannot gain any way other than living through them; they may want to share their experiences and knowledge, they want to help others, and they want to know that their lives have meaning. Seeing these people only for their physical needs means seeing only a fraction of the whole, and in what is lost the nurse misses the true person.

As a student, you will meet older people in many placements. You can learn a lot from these placements – physical skilled nursing care is just one small part. Learn to listen, and learn to learn from your patients. Learn about their lives, and the history they have experienced. Comfort them, talk about the loved ones they have lost, and learn about your own life in the process. Very few conversations can be as rewarding as one held with an older person reminiscing about special times in his or her life.

The opportunities for health promotion and rehabilitation cannot be minimized – and should not be missed. The care of the older person is more than incontinence and dementia; it is about promoting independence, good health and patient involvement, health education and holism in partnership with the older person. It's about supporting someone in mind, body and spirit. The skills you learn caring for older people are not only useful; they also underpin all the nursing you will ever do. If you can listen, see people not for their limits but for their potential, have empathy and understanding, and deliver skilled care with patience, kindness and compassion, then you will offer the best in nursing care.

Knowledge and Skills Framework

Every person's job in the NHS will have a Knowledge and Skills Framework (KSF) outline. This outline is linked to the job description and outlines the skills employees are expected to have to do their job.

The NHS KSF, on which the development review process is based, is designed to:

- identify the knowledge and skills that individuals need to do their job
- guide staff development
- provide a way to assess and review staff skill and development
- provide a basis for progression in pay based on increasing skills and responsibilities.

The KSF is made up of 30 dimensions. These dimensions are grouped into themes, and outline the functions required to provide a good-quality service to the public across all the levels and groups of staff. Six of the dimensions are core, which means that they are relevant to every post in the NHS. The **core dimensions** are:

1. Communication
2. Personal and people development
3. Health, safety and security
4. Service improvement
5. Quality
6. Equality and diversity.

The other 24 dimensions are specific – they apply to some, but not all, jobs in the NHS. These are grouped into themes:

- Health and well-being: looking at care, assessment and treatment
- Estates and facilities: looking at equipment, environments, transport, vehicles and logistics
- Information and knowledge: looking at IT, information processes (information collection and analysis) and information/knowledge resources

- General: looking at learning and development, development and innovation, procurement and commissioning, financial management, services and project management, people management, capacity and capability, and public relations and marketing.

Each of the dimensions has level descriptors from 1 to 4. These descriptors describe the level at which the person should function: 1 is usually very limited to either being told what to do or having no judgement or input, and 4 means having responsibility across wide parts of an organization or service.

The KSF also has gateways – points at which you have to prove that you have met certain requirements to proceed. To use an example: newly qualified nurses are at Band 5 Step One for the first 6 months of their career; after 6 months in post and a period of successful preceptorship, they move up to the next increment. This reflects the growth and development present in the job, and the KSF, in the first 6 months. At later stages in the band there are additional gateways past which nurses cannot progress until there have been accomplishments or achievements that reflect excellence and skill.

The other use of the KSF is identifying what help and support the nurse needs to advance. If you have a responsibility in the KSF to assess patients, for example, and you have no idea what that means, you need to start thinking about how to gain assessment skills: do you need a course, preceptorship or self-directed study? You and your manager make a plan, and your manager supports you.

In addition to the title and indicators, there are examples of application. Your manager has to provide applications that fit the kind of work you do. The KSF plays a critical part in relating to actual jobs through the development of a 'post outline', an outline with the dimensions and the applications expected for particular jobs in areas of an organization. Your job outline should include the core dimensions, as well as two or three other dimensions. Many of the core dimensions cover a significant amount, so if you have a lot of dimensions look at what they are asking you to do to apply them (areas of application) and see if they don't fit under the core dimensions.

There are other areas of the Agenda for Change that will continue to evolve and change – although the KSF is relatively stable, it still may change.

At the time of writing there are several important issues and events that may impact on the KSF. These include the following:

- For some years, hospitals in England have been encouraged to become Foundation Trusts if they meet specific quality and financial management criteria. They continue to remain within the NHS and must work within NHS guidance and standards but have more operational and financial independence in how they are run. All NHS trusts are expected to become Foundation Trusts by 2013–2014 (Holme 2013).

- Many changes in the NHS structure in England following the Health and Social Care Act 2012, such as the creation of clinically-led commissioning to replace the Primary Care Trusts (PCTs).

- Discussion around Local and Regional pay scales.
- The development of new posts, such as assistant practitioners.
- Last but not least, the current financial climate and government spending controls.

Given the pace of changes, readers are advised to keep up to date with events by accessing reliable media sources and nursing journals, such as the *Nursing Standard* and *Nursing Times*.

REFERENCES

Health and Social Care Act 2012 Online. Available at www.dh.gov.uk/health/2012/06/act-explained

Holmes, A., 2013. Health and social care delivery systems. In: Brooker, C., Waugh, A., (Eds.), 2013. Foundation of Nursing Practice. Fundamentals of Holistic Care, second ed. Mosby, Edinburgh

Appendix 8
Root Words, Prefixes and Suffixes

ROOT WORDS

Root word	Meaning	Example
acou	hearing	acoustic
acr	extremities, height	acrodynia
aden	gland	adenitis
aer	air	aerobic
algesi	pain	algesia
andr	male	androgens
angi	vessel, duct	angioplasty
ankyl	crooked, stiff, bent	ankylosis
arter	artery	arteriosclerosis
arthr	joint	arthropathy
articul	joint	articulation
atel	imperfect, incomplete	atelectasis
ather	yellowish, fatty plaque	atheroma
aur	ear	aural
aut	self	autoantigen
axill	armpit	axilla
bil	bile	bilirubin
blast	developing cell	blastoderm
blephar	eyelid	blepharon
brachi	arm	brachial cyst
bronch	bronchus	bronchitis
bucc	cheek	buccal cavity
carcin	cancer	carcinogen
cardi, coron	heart	cardiac, coronary
caud	tail	cauda equina
celi	abdomen	celiocolpotomy
ceph, cephal	head	cephalocele

Root word	Meaning	Example
cerv	neck (like neck of a bottle)	cervix
cheil	lip	cheilosis
chole	gall, bile	cholestasis
chondr	cartilage	chondritis
chrom	colour	chromatopsia
cortic	outer layer of an organ	cortical
cost	rib	costal cartilage
crani	head	craniodidymus
crani	skull	cranium
cry	cold	cryoanalgesia
crypt	hidden	cryptomenorrhoea
cutane	skin	cutaneous
cyan	blue	cyanosis
cyst	bladder, sac	cystectomy
cyt, cyte	cell	cytology
dacry	tear, tear duct	dacryocystitis
dactyl	fingers or toes	dactylology
dent	tooth	dentine
derm	skin	dermis
dermat	skin	dermatology
dextr	right	dextral
dipl	double	diplopia
dips	thirst	dipsogen
dynam	power or strength	dyamometer
ectop	located away from usual place	ectopia vesicae
electr	electricity, electrical activity	electroysis
encephal	brain	encephalitis
entera	entrails (guts)	enteral
esthesi	sensation, feeling	anaesthesia
eti	cause (of disease)	aetiology
faci	face, covering	facial
gastr	stomach	gastric
gloss	tongue	glossitis
gluc	sweetness, sugar	glucose
glycos	sugar	glycosuria
gynae	woman	gynaecoid
haem	blood	haemorrhage
hepa, hepat	liver	hepatitis
heter	other	heterogenous
hist	tissue	histopathogy

Root word	Meaning	Example
homo	same, unchanging	homozygous
hydr	water	hydration
hypn	sleep	hypnosis
irid	iris	iridectomy
isch	deficiency	ischaemia
kal	potassium	hypokalaemia
kerat	hard tissue	keratin
kinesi	motion, movement	bradykinesia
labi	lips	labia
lacrim	tears, tear duct	lacrimal
lact	milk	lactose
lapar	abdomen	laparotomy
later	side	lateral
leuk	white	leukaemia
lingu	tongue	lingual
lip	fat	lipid
lith	stone	lithotripsy
mamm, mast	breast	mammogram, mastitis
mandibu	lower jaw	mandibular
maxil	upper jaw	maxilla
meatus	opening	meatal
melan	black	melanosis
ment	mind, thinking	mental
metr	uterus	metrorrhagia
mono	one	monoamine
morph	form	morphology
my, myos	muscle	myoma, myositis
myc	fungus	mycelium
myel	bone marrow, spinal cord	myelocytes, myelitis
myelon	bone marrow	myelonic
myo, musculo	muscle	myocardium, musculoskeletal
myring	eardrum	myringotomy
nas	nose	nasal
nat	birth	natal
necr	death, dead	necrophila, necrosis
nephr, ren	kidney	nephron, renal
neur	nerve	neural
neuro	nerve	neuroblastoma
noct	night	nocturia
ocu	eye	ocular

Root word	Meaning	Example
olig	few	oligohydramnios
onc	tumour	oncology
onych	nail	onycholysis
oo, ov	egg, ovum	oocyte, ova
ophth	vision, the eye	ophthalmoscope
orch, orchid	testis, testicle	orchitis, orchidectomy
orth	straight	orthopaedic
oste	bone	osteon
ot	ear	otitis
ox	oxygen	oxyhaemoglobin
pachy	thick	pachyderma
part	birth	parturition
path	disease	pathophysiology
pector	chest	pectoralis major
pelv	pelvis, pelvic bone	pelvimeter
phag	eat, swallow	phagocyte
phas	speech	aphasia
phleb	vein	phlebitis
phot	light	photophobia
phren	mind, diaphragm	phrenology, phrenic
plasm	plasma, in the blood	plasmin, plasmapheresis
pneumo, pnoea	air, lung	pneumonia, dyspnoea
pod	foot	podiatrist
poster	back (of body)	posterior
pseud	fake, false	pseudomembranous
psych	mind	psychiatry
py	pus	pyuria
pyr	fever, heat	pyrexia
quadr	four	quadriceps
rhin	nose	rhinoplasty
sarc	flesh, connective tissue	sarcoma
scoli	crooked, curved	scoliosis
sept	septum	septate
septum	division, wall	septal
sinus	empty space	sinusitis
som	the body	soma
somat	body	somatostatin
somn	sleep	somnambulism
spir	breath, breathe, breathing	inspire, respiration, spirometry
splen	spleen	splenectomy

Root word	Meaning	Example
spondyl	vertebra(e), spine, spinal or vertebral column	spondylitis
stoma	mouth, an opening	stomatitis, stomal
therm	heat	thermogenesis
thorac	thorax (chest)	thoracic
thromb	clot	thrombus
tom	cut, section	tomography
top	place, outside	topography
tymp	drum	tympanic
ungu	nail	unguis
ure, uri	urine	urethra, urinary
vas	vascular, veins, duct	vasoactive, vas deferens
vesi-	pouch, sac	vesicle, vesiculitis

PREFIXES

Prefix	Meaning	Example
a-, an-	without, missing	aplasia, anaemia
ab-	from, away from	abductor
ad-	to, toward	adduct
ambi-	both	ambidextrous
ante-	before	antenatal
anti-	against	antiviral
bi-, bin-	two	biceps, binaural
brady-	slow	bradycardia
chlor-	green	chloropsia
circum-	around	circumduction
con-	together	concrescence
contra-	against	contraception
cyan-	blue	cyanopsia
de-	take way, reduce	decompression
dia-	complete, through	diameter, diapedesis
dis-	undo, take away from	dislocate
dys-	difficult, abnormal	dysuria
ecto-	outside	ectoderm
endo-	inside	endoderm
epi-	on, over, covering	epidermis
erythr-	red	erythrocyte

Prefix	Meaning	Example
eu-	normal, good	eustress
ex-, exo-	outside	exogenous
extra-	outside of	extracellular
hemi-	half	hemianopia
hetero-	different	heterozygous
homo-	same	homograft
hyper-	above, in excess	hypertension
hypo-	below, deficient	hypocalcaemia
in-, im-	not,	inappetence
infra-	underneath, below	infraorbital
inter-	between	intercostal
intra-	inside	intramuscular
jaun-	yellow	jaundice
leuk/o-, leuc/o-	white	leukocidins, leucocyte
macro-	large	macrophage
mal-	bad, abnormal	malnutrition
melan-	black	melanoma
meso-	middle, medium	mesoderm
meta-	change	metabolize
micro-	small	microglia
mono-	one	monoclonal
multi-	many	multigravida
neo-	new	neoplasm
pan-	all	pandemic
para-	next to, around, beyond	paracrine
per-	through	percutaneous
peri-	surrounding	perimenopause
poly-	many	polycystic
post-	after	postmortem
pre-, pro-	before	premenopausal
pseudo-	fake	pseudocyst
purpur-	purple	purpura
quad-	four	quadriceps
re-	back, again	reflux
retro-	behind	retrograde
rube-	red	rubor
semi-	half	semiprone
sub-	under, beneath	subdural
super-, supra-	over, above	superinfection, suprarenal

Prefix	Meaning	Example
sym-, syn-	together, joined	symphysis, synechia
tachy-	fast	tachycardia
trans-	through, across	transcutaneous
tri-	three	tricuspid
ultra-	above, beyond, extra	ultrasound
uni-	one	uniovular

SUFFIXES

Suffix	Meaning	Example
-aemia, -emia	blood	polycythaemia
-algia	pain	neuralgia
-cele	hernia, swelling	hydrocele
-centesis	tap, puncture	paracentesis
-clasia	crushing, to break down	osteoclasia
-desis	binding, stabilization	arthrodesis
-dynia	pain, swelling, discomfort	pleurodynia
-ectasis	dilation, expansion	telangiectasis
-ectomy	removal	pneumonectomy
-gen	beginning	pepsinogen
-gram	record of data	electrocardiogram
-graph	instrument for recording	electrocardiograph
-graphy	act of recording data	encephalography
-ia	an unhealthy state	hypoxia
-iac	indicates person has certain conditions	cardiac
-iasis	abnormal condition, presence of	myiasis
-icle	small	ossicle
-ism	condition, state of being	prostatism
-ist	a specialist	gynaecologist
-itis	inflammation	sinusitis
-lysis	loosen, destruction	glycolysis
-malacia	softening	osteomalacia
-megaly	enlargement	acromegaly
-meter	instrument for measuring	thermometer
-metry	measurement of	telemetry
-oid	resemble	android

Suffix	Meaning	Example
-ole	small	arteriole
-oma	tumour, swelling	carcinoma
-osis	abnormal condition	psychosis
-pathy	disease	retinopathy
-penia	decrease, deficiency	thrombocytopenia
-pexy	fixation, suspension	orchidopexy
-phagia	eating, swallowing	odynophagia
-phasia	speech	paraphasia
-phobia	fear	zoophobia
-plasty	formation, repair	keratoplasty
-plegia	paralysis	hemiplegia
-ptosis	prolapse, drooping	nephroptosis
-rrhage	burst forth	haemorrhage
-rrhaphy	suture	colporrhaphy
-rrhoea	discharge	diarrhoea
-rrhexis	rupture	karyorrhexis
-sclerosis	hardening	atherosclerosis
-scope	instrument for viewing	cystoscope
-scopy	examination	colposcopy
-spasm	involuntary contraction, twitching	vasospasm
-stomy	forming an opening	ileostomy
-tomy	incision, to cut into	thoracotomy
-tripsy	to crush	lithotripsy
-ule	small	pustule
-y	condition, process	itchy

The following are special suffixes that show singular and plural endings.

Singular	Plural
-a	ae
-ax	aces
-en	ina
-ix/-ex	ices
-sis	ses
-on	a
-um	a
-us	i
-y	ies
-ma	mata

REFERENCES

Cohen B 1998 Medical Terminology – An Illustrated Guide. Lippincott- Raven Publishers, Philadelphia, PA

Gyls B, Wedding M 2004 Medical Terminology: A Systems Approach, 4th edn. Lippincott, Williams & Wilkins, Philadelphia, PA

Hutton AR 2006 An Introduction to Medical Terminology for Health Care, 4th edn. Churchill Livingstone, Edinburgh

Appendix 9
Normal Values

BLOOD (HAEMATOLOGY)

Test	Reference range
Activated partial thromboplastin time (APTT)	30–40 s
Bleeding time (Ivy)	2–8 min
Erythrocyte sedimentation rate (ESR):	
Adult women	3–15 mm/h
Adult men	1–10 mm/h
Fibrinogen	1.5–4.0 g/l
Folate (serum)	4–18 mcg/l (µg/l)
Haemoglobin:	
Women	115–165 g/l (11.5–16.5 g/dl)
Men	130–180 g/l (13–18 g/dl)
Haptoglobins	0.3–2.0 g/l
Mean cell haemoglobin (MCH)	27–32 pg
Mean cell haemoglobin concentration (MCHC)	30–35 g/dl
Mean cell volume (MCV)	78–95 fl
Packed cell volume (PCV or haematocrit):	
Women	0.35–0.47 (35–47%)
Men	0.40–0.54 (40–54%)
Platelets (thrombocytes)	150–400 × 10^9/l
Prothrombin time	12–16 s
Red cells (erythrocytes):	
Women	3.8–5.3 × 10^{12}/l
Men	4.5–6.5 × 10^{12}/l
Reticulocytes (newly formed red cells in adults)	25–85 × 10^9/l
White cells total (leucocytes)	4.0–11.0 × 10^9/l

BLOOD – VENOUS PLASMA (BIOCHEMISTRY)

Test	Reference range
Alanine aminotransferase (ALT)	10–40 U/l
Albumin	36–47 g/l
Alkaline phosphatase	40–125 U/l
Amylase	<100 U/l
Aspartate aminotransferase (AST)	10–45 U/l
Bicarbonate (arterial)	22–28 mmol/l
Bilirubin (total)	2–17 µmol/l
Caeruloplasmin	0.2–0.6 g/l
Calcium	2.1–2.6 mmol/l
Chloride	95–105 mmol/l
Cholesterol (total)	Ideally below 5.2 mmol/l
HDL cholesterol	>1.0 mmol/l
$PaCO_2$ (arterial)	4.4–6.1 kPa
Copper	13–24 µmol/l
Cortisol (at 0800 h)	160–565 nmol/l
Creatine kinase (total):	
Women	30–135 U/l
Men	55–170 U/l
Creatinine	55–120 µmol/l
Gamma-glutamyl transferase (GGT):	
Women	5–35 U/l
Men	10–55 U/l
Globulins	24–37 g/l
Glucose (venous blood, fasting)	3.6–5.8 mmol/l
Glycosylated haemoglobin (HbA_{1c})	4.0–6.0%
Hydrogen ion concentration (arterial)	35–44 nmol/l
Iron:	
Women	10–28 µmol/l
Men	14–32 µmol/l
Iron-binding capacity total (TIBC)	45–70 µmol/l
Lactate (arterial)	0.3–1.4 mmol/l
Lactate dehydrogenase (total)	230–460 U/l

Test	Reference range
Lead (adults, whole blood)	$< 1.7\,\mu mol/l$
Magnesium	0.7–1.0 mmol/l
Osmolality	275–290 mmol/kg
PaO_2 (arterial)	12–15 kPa
Oxygen saturation (arterial)	>97%
pH	7.36–7.42
Phosphate (fasting)	0.8–1.4 mmol/l
Potassium (serum)	3.6–5.0 mmol/l
Protein (total)	60–80 g/l
Sodium	136–145 mmol/l
Transferrin	2–4 g/l
Triglycerides (fasting)	0.6–1.8 mmol/l
Urate:	
Women	0.12–0.36 mmol/l
Men	0.12–0.42 mmol/l
Urea	2.5–6.5 mmol/l
Uric acid:	
Women	0.09–0.36 mmol/l
Men	0.1–0.45 mmol/l
Vitamin A	$0.7–3.5\,\mu mol/l$
Vitamin C	$23–57\,\mu mol/l$
Zinc	$11–22\,\mu mol/l$

CEREBROSPINAL FLUID

Test	Reference range
Cells	$<5 \times 10^6$ cells/l (all mononuclear)
Chloride	120–170 mmol/l
Glucose	2.5–4.0 mmol/l
Pressure (adult)	50–180 mm/H_2O
Protein	100–400 mg/l

URINE

Test	Reference range
Albumin/creatinine ratio (ACR)	< 3.5 mg albumin/mmol creatinine
Calcium (normal diet)	up to 7.5 mmol/24 h
Copper	Up to 0.6 μmol/24 h
Cortisol (24 h collection)	25–250 nmol/24 h
Creatinine	9–20 mmol/24 h
5–Hydroxyindole–3–acetic acid (5HIAA)	10–45 μmol/24 h
Magnesium	3.3–5.0 mmol/24 h
Oxalate	0.04–0.49 mmol/24 h
pH	4–8
Phosphate	15–50 mmol/24 h
Porphyrins (total)	90–370 nmol/24 h
Potassium (depends on intake)	25–100 mmol/24 h
Protein (total)	no more than 0.3 g/l
Sodium (depends on intake)	100–200 mmol/24 h
Urea	170–500 mmol/24 h

FAECES

Test	Reference range
Fat content (daily output on normal diet)	< 7 g/24 h
Fat (as stearic acid)	11–18 mmol/24 h

Index

A

7 rights, medication administration 133
Abdellah, F.G. 43–4
'academic style' 61
academic work 54–69
ACCESS model of transcultural nursing 43–5
  Abdellah's 21 problems 43–4
accountability 192
ACT A PUP mnemonic 81
activities of daily life 39–40
adult nurse 13
advance statement (advance directive) 197
Agenda for change 16–17, 229
Aldridge, J. 45
anatomy, positions/descriptions 127–30
assertiveness 100–4
  confrontations 101–4
  defined 100
  personal 101
assessment
  of patient 39, 41
  self-assessment 50–1
assignments
  assignment brief 58
  deadlines 222
  tutorials 60, 64
assignments (writing assignments) 58
  answering the question 59–60
  backing up 63
  feedback and notes 64
  information worksheet 68
  and patient privacy 65
  preparation 63
  structuring 60–1
  time frame 62
assistant, health care assistant (HCA) 16, 22
audits 156–7

B

back injury 189
banding 17
becoming a nurse 18–22
Benner, Patricia 37
  nursing theory 37

biohazard materials 189
blood, normal values 240–2
body language 97–9
Bolam test, negligence 194
boundaries 104–5
  good 104–5
  secrets 104
Boykin and Schoenhofer: nursing as caring 47
branches of nursing 72–3
  relationship with others 83
  transfering to other branches 84
British National Formulary (BNF) 132
bullying 194–5, 201

C

capacity
  and consent 196
  Mental Capacity Act (2005) 195–6
Casey, A. 44
  model of nursing 44
cerebrospinal fluid, normal values 242–3
character, and fitness-to-practise 193
cheating (plagiarism) 57
child health models 44, 48
children's nurses 13
children's nursing 224–5
client care plans, learning disability nursing 218–19
clinical audit 156
clinical placement coordinator 83
clinical placements 69–89
  advance visits 74
  checklist 87–8
  overseas 73
  patient perspectives 75
  patients' rights 73
  placement checklist 87–8
  pre-registration nurse education 71–2
  preparation for visit 74
  problems 77–9
  supernumerary status 79–81
clinical skills 201
  essential skills clusters 211–12
clinical tutor/clinical educator 84
Code of Practice (May 2008) 9

common foundation programme 202
communication skills 93–7, 228
   improving communication 95–7
community psychiatric nurses
      (CPNs) 16
competence, decision-making 191
competency framework 210–11
computers 66–7
confidentiality 64–5
consent 190–1
   and capacity 196
   doctor's assessment 196
   Mental Capacity Act (2005) 195–6
conversions (maths) 142
Coolidge, Calvin *quoted* 200
'cracking the code' 123–30
criminal convictions 19

D

Data Protection Act (1998) 186–7
Defining Nursing (RCN) 32
delegation 108–10
   priorities 108
   what to delegate 109–10
depression 106–7
diary 24
disabilities 26, 183–6
   dignity, respect 185
   legal guardian 191
   misperceptions 19, 184–6
   students with 4
   see also learning disability nursing
Disability Discrimination Act (NI) 19, 183
disability rights officer 186
disclosure of mistakes 219
doctrine of necessity 197
Donaldson, Sir Liam 119–20
dosage calculations 141–3
   conversions (maths) 142
   quiz 145–52
dress and appearance 73–4, 220
drugs *see* medication administration
drugs, recreational 193
duty of care 189
   negligence 193
dyscalculia 138
dyslexia 19

E

Ecology of Health Model 45
education, changes 70
elderly people 226–7
entry requirements, universities 18

environmental factors, Roper model 41
Equality Act (GB) 19, 183
Equality and Human Rights Commission
      in Britain 26
essence of care 121–2
essential skills clusters 211–12
ethics 112–16
   advocacy 115
   asking for help 115
   difficult decisions 115
   do no harm/do good 113
   ethical issues 160, 202
   justice and fairness 113
   personal philosophies 114–15
   personal prejudices 114
   respect 113–14
   trust, truth-telling and honesty 113
European Computer Driving Licence
      (ECDL) 66
evidence-based practice 153
expressed consent 190

F

family-based care 36
'final thoughts' 199–200
fitness-to-practise 192–4
   hearings 9
Fitzpatrick's rhythm model 45–6
forensic nursing 15
   Psychology of Criminal Conduct 221
forensic service 220
Foundation Trusts 229
funding arrangements 20–1

G

Gibbs (1988) model of reflection 173
governance 117, 119–21
   clinical 119–21
guardian, legal 191

H

haematology, normal values 240–2
harassment 194–5
health care assistant (HCA) 16, 22
health promotion 203
Health and Safety at Work Act (1974)
      187–8
   employees' obligations 188
   employers' obligations 187
Health and Social Care Act (2012) 229
health visitors 13

Henderson, Virginia 31–2
  nursing defined 2, 31, 39
hoisting equipment 220
holism/holistic care 33–5
  defined 34–5
  empathy 34
  NMC Code of Professional Conduct
    (NMC 2002) 33
  nursing models 35
  respect 34
  sensitivity 34
  understanding 34
Human Resources (Personnel)
  department 22

I

implied consent 190
information
  check with patient 187
  Data Protection Act 186–7
  personal 64
  for portfolio 187
  sensitive 64
  staff 187
informed consent 191
informed refusal (of care) 191
IT skills 66–7

J

Johns (1994) model of reflection 173
journals 158–9, 206

K

King, I.M. 46
King's model 46
Knowledge and Skills Framework (KSF)
  16, 228–30

L

language, medical jargon 124–6
leadership 116–18
  importance of 117
  make things better 116
  NHS Plan (DH 2000) 116
learning in the clinical environment
  203
Learning Disabilities: Towards Inclusion
  (ed. Atherton and Crickmore)
  221

learning disability nursing 13, 216–23
  1990 Act 217
  becoming qualified 221
  client care plans 218–19
  Ecology of Health Model 45
  history 216–17
  local trust policies 219
  role of nurse 218–19
  see also mental health nursing
legal issues 180–98, 203
Leininger
  M. 46
  Transcultural Nursing Model 46
Levine, conservation model 46
library, personal 24
lifespan defined 40
link tutor 84
listening 98–9
literature review 159

M

Making a Difference 71–2
manual-handling policy 189
maths
  cheat sheet 139
  conversions 142
  dosage calculations 141–3
  hints and tips 141
  self-test 140
  weight and volume 143
matron 16
medical jargon 124–6
medical terminology 126–9
medication administration 131–7
  7 rights 133–6
  dosage calculations 141–3
  errors 131–2
  numeracy 138–41
  numeracy quiz 145–52
  special considerations 137
  summary 137
Mental Capacity Act (2005) 195–6
Mental Health Act 1983 221
mental health nursing 13–14, 212–15
  models 48
  see also learning disability nursing
mentorship 81–3
  duties/functions 82
  relationship with mentor 74–5
midwifery studies 12, 13
military nursing students 22
misconduct 9
mistakes, disclosure 219
models of nursing 37–52
models and theories 203

N

Narayanasamy, A. 43
national audits 157
National Union of Students 207–8
negligence 193–4
  Bolam test 194
Neuman's model of nursing 46–7
NHS Business Services Authority 20
NHS and Community Care Act (1990) 217
NHS Plan (DH 2000), leadership 116
NICE, macro vs micro application 165
Nightingale's environmental adaptation
    model 47
NMC see Nursing and Midwifery Council
    (NMC)
normal values 240–3
  blood 240–2
  cerebrospinal fluid 242
  faeces 243
  urine 243
normalization 220
  and social role valorization 217
norms 118–19
  good maintenance of 118–19
Nottingham model 44–5
numeracy 138–41
  cheat sheet 139
  quiz 145–52
  see also maths
nurse
  'Access course' 20
  aptitude for becoming a 18–19
  basic minimum qualification 20
  becoming a 18–22
  degree course 20
  past experience 20
  resident in UK 21
  vs student, public perceptions 189–90
nurse appearance/behaviour
  holiday dreams 76–7
  jewellery 74
  long hair and fingernails 74
  punctuality 74
  standards of dress and appearance
      73–4, 220
  to staff 75
nurse auxiliary 16
nurse consultant 15
nurse education, changes 70
nurse manager 16
nurse practitioner 15
nursing
  basic branches 12
  as a career 5
  course funding arrangements 20
  defined 2, 31–2

nursing (Continued)
  fields 210
  philosophy (principles) 35–6
  pre-registration standards 3
  purpose/domain/focus/intervention 31–2
  students with disabilities 4
  value base 32
  Vocation vs profession 3
nursing basics 89–99
  basic nursing qualities 89–90
  body language 97–9
  communication skills 93–7
  interpreting patients' fears 94–5
  listening 98–9
  nurse vs patient attitudes 90–3
  positive non-threatening
      communication 93
  process 32–3, 37
  verbal communication 94–7
nursing language
  introduction 123–4
  medical jargon 124–6
Nursing Law and Ethics (Tingle and Cribb)
    221
Nursing and Midwifery Council (NMC)
    5–8, 210–12
  Code of Professional Conduct 7
  contacts 26–7
  Guide for Students of Nursing and
      Midwifery 7
  guidelines for student nurses 219–20
  personal identification number (PIN) 8
nursing models 37–52
  commitment to partnership 32
  defined 38–9
  framework defined 37
nursing practice 204
nursing process 32–3
  assess 33
  evaluate 33
  implement 33
  plan 33
  theory 37
Nursing Qualifications pre-2007 11
Nursing Standard 177
Nursing Times, portfolio development
    178

O

O'Brien, John, 'five service
    accomplishments' 217
older people 226–7
Orem: self-care deficit model 48
organization 110–12
  priorities 110–12
overseas clinical placements 73

P

parent–staff interaction model,
    paediatric Care 48
patient privacy, and written assignments
    65
patients' rights 73
Peach Report (Fitness for Practice UKCC
    1999) 70–1
Peplau: interpersonal relations model 48
persistence 199–200
personal identification number (PIN) 8
philosophy (principles) 35–6
placements 176
plagiarism 56–7
portfolios 175–9
    development 177–8
    post-registration education and
        practice (PREP) 177–8
    student portfolio 176
pre-placement visit 189
pre-registration nurse education 71–2
    standards 3, 210–12
prefixes 126–7, 235–7
PREP Handbook 177
Primary Care Trusts (PCTs) 229
prison nurse 15
Professional Practice and Registration
    Committee 72
Project 2000 70
psychological factors, Roper model 40
Public Health Practitioners 11

Q

Quality Assurance Agency (QAA) 23

R

records/record-keeping 181–3
    abbreviations 181
    corrections 182
    counter-signature 182
    good (NMC) 182–3
    objective and non-judgemental 182
referencing, checking the references 55, 163
reflective journal 175
reflective models 173–4
    Gibbs (1988) 173
    Johns (1994) 173
reflective practice 171–9, 204
    defined 171
    examples 172
    importance to practice 174–5
    summary 178
refusal (to give consent) 197

register (NMC)
    categories 10
    levels 10
Registration process 8
research 153–70, 204
    application: macro vs micro
        165–6
    applying research to practice 163
    clinical audit 156
    quantitative vs qualitative research
        155–6
    reading 157
    research article 164–5
research article
    abstract and key words 159, 168
    acknowledgements 163
    author and title 158, 168
    data collection 161
    ethical issues 160
    introduction 159, 168
    literature review 159, 169
    method and sample 160, 169–70
    read for relevance and usefulness
        166
    referencing 163
    results/discussion 162, 170
    summary 162
    validity/reliability/rigour 161
research committee 167
research proposal 166–7
    answering questions 167
    common mistakes 170
    downloadable form 168–70
research statements 157
researching placement area 74
Rogers: unitary healthcare model 49
root words, suffixes and prefixes 126–7,
        231–9
    prefixes 235–7
    root words 231–5
    suffixes 237–9
Roper, Nancy 38
Roper model 30, 38–43
    activities of daily life 39–40
        influencing factors 40–1
    assessment of patient 39, 41
    biological factors 40
    dependence/independence
        continuum 40
    environmental factors 41
    evaluation 42–3
    implementation techniques 42
    individuality in living 41
    lifespan defined 40
    planning (coping with problems)
        41–2
    politico-economic 41
    psychological factors 40
    role of nurse 41–3

Roper model *(Continued)*
  sociocultural factors 40–1
  transcultural care 35
Roy: adaptive model 50
Royal College of Nursing, nursing
    defined 2

S

safety issues 188–9
  see also Health and Safety at Work Act
      (1974)
school nurse 15
search engines 67
searching skills 67
self-assessment 50–1
sensitivity 34, 75
service evaluation 157
sharps disposal/policy 188
signature 182
skills
  clinical skills 201, 211–12
  communication skills 93–7
  IT skills 66–7
  searching skills 67
  study skills 205
skills clusters 211–12
smoking 177
social policy 205
social role valorization, and
    normalization 217
standards 121–2
  fitness-to-practise hearings 9
Standards for Better Health (S48H) 122
stereotyping 34–5
stress 106–8
  coping strategies 107–8
  depression 106–7
  negative and positive solutions 106
student finance 21–2
students with disabilities 4

study skills 205
suffixes 130, 237–9
supernumerary status, defined 79–81
support workers, and NMC 6

T

teachers 83–4
Tippex 182
'tools of the trade' 100–22
traffic offences 193
transcultural care 35
  nursing model 46
tutorials 60, 64

U

uniform, standards of dress and
    appearance 73–4, 220
union, joining 26
United Kingdom Central Council (UKCC) 7
universities
  entry requirements 18
  information 22–4
unprofessional behaviour 65
urine, normal values 243

V

verbal communication 94–7

W

Watson: theory of caring 50
wesites 21
whistle-blowing 220
word root basics 129–30
writing an assignment 58